Simplified drugs
and solutions for nurses
INCLUDING MATHEMATICS

Simplified drugs and solutions for nurses
INCLUDING MATHEMATICS

NORMA DISON, R.N., B.A., M.A., M.S.

Assistant Professor, Medical Surgical Nursing,
Winona State University,
Winona, Minnesota

EIGHTH EDITION

with **18** illustrations

The C. V. Mosby Company

ST. LOUIS   TORONTO   1984

MOSBY

A TRADITION OF PUBLISHING EXCELLENCE

Editor: **Julie Cardamon**
Assistant editor: **Bess Arends**
Manuscript editor: **Roger McWilliams**
Design: **Staff**
Production: **Carol O'Leary, Mary Stueck, Barbara Merritt**

EIGHTH EDITION

Printed in the United States of America

The C.V. Mosby Company
11830 Westline Industrial Drive, St. Louis, Missouri 63146

Library of Congress Cataloging in Publication Data

Dison, Norma Greenler.
  Simplified drugs and solutions for nurses, including mathematics.

  1. Pharmaceutical arithmetic—Problems, exercises,
etc. 2. Drugs—Dosage—Problems, exercises, etc.
I. Title. [DNLM: 1. Drugs—Administration and dosage—
Nursing texts. 2. Mathematics—Nursing texts. QV 16
D611s]
RS57.N37 1984   615'.4'01513   83-8301
ISBN 0-8016-1313-2

C/VH/VH 9 8 7 6 5 4 3 2 1   03/C/342

PREFACE

This edition of *Simplified Drugs and Solutions for Nurses, Including Mathematics* has been revised in keeping with current practices and the suggestions of readers. The purpose of this book is still to emphasize basic arithmetic skills needed by nurses to solve problems involving dosages and solutions.

All of the chapters have been carefully reviewed and updated. New problems have been added to the exercises following each chapter. The arithmetic pretest has been rearranged so that the content is in the same sequence as the text content. A new chapter on computing fractions, decimals, and percentages has been added. Parts of some chapters have been rewritten to clarify the presentation of material. Problems dealing with U-80 insulin and corresponding syringes have been deleted, since the manufacture of this insulin has been discontinued in the United States.

In keeping with the different styles of learning, several methods are given for solving each type of problem. The first method shows how to relate the problem to information found on the label of the drug to be administered; the second shows how to establish a proportion to solve the problem; and the third provides a formula into which known variables are substituted before working the problem. The student is encouraged to decide which method is most acceptable in terms of individual ability and to apply this method consistently in the solution of the problems.

I recognize that methods of measurement other than metric are encountered less frequently today than in the past. The decision to retain problems involving conversion from one system of measurement to another is based on knowledge that such converting continues to be necessary.

Appreciation is extended to the many readers who sent helpful comments and suggestions.

Norma Dison

CONTENTS

INTRODUCTION

Nurses are given considerable responsibility for the care of patients when they are allowed to prepare and administer medications. Nurses who perform such tasks assume legal, moral, and ethical responsibilities as well. The nurse must know how the prescribed drugs are expected to affect the patient and his condition, their usual range of dosage, their route of administration, precautions to be followed in their administration, and signs and symptoms of side effects. The nurse must also teach the patient and the family about the medications that are to be continued in the home; this requires creativity, patience, and repetition of information along with opportunities for the patient to practice administering his own medication.

The basic arithmetic used in daily living and taught in elementary school is used in calculating dosages and in making solutions. Review and practice facilitate the basic processes used in solving the problems of drugs and solutions. The first part of this book reviews basic arithmetic, the second part presents different systems of measurement and conversion from one system of measurement to another, and the last section presents different types of problems that may be encountered. When working problems that require converting from one system of measurement to another, answers that differ from each other by as much as 10% may result. An amount greater than this is certain to be in error. In problems that do not require conversion from one system of measurement to another, no margin of error is permitted. It must be remembered that an answer is either right or wrong when working problems that involve drugs and solutions.

In addition to having considerable knowledge about the drug and the patient, the nurse also rechecks the order, drug preparation, and dose carefully during its preparation and checks again whenever a patient questions whether a medication is the correct one. These practices help ensure the safety of the patient. If the nurse has doubts or questions about a medication, dose, or calculation, it is wise to ask another nurse or the supervisor to also check. The pharmacist is an excellent resource person to consult when questions arise about medications, and the physician is consulted when there are questions about the order for medications.

Hospital policies concerning administration of medications vary. Those hospitals that have in-service training for new employees may not allow nurses to administer medications until they have completed the unit on medications and have undergone appropriate supervision. It is good policy to have a registered nurse available to assist and supervise practical (vocational) nurses if the agency allows them to administer medications.

I BASIC ARITHMETIC

ARITHMETIC PRETEST

EXPLANATION: The following pretest may be used to determine the areas in which arithmetic review is needed. After completing the pretest and checking the answers, it is suggested that the individual analyze the reasons for each error made. Chapters 1 through 15 review the arithmetic processes used to work the problems on the pretest.

I. Express in Roman numerals:

1. 14 _____   4. 100 _____   7. 38 _____

2. 25 _____   5. 13 _____   8. 19 _____

3. 57 _____   6. 44 _____   9. 5 _____

II. Express in Arabic numbers:

1. CX _____   4. XXIX _____   7. XXV _____

2. VI _____   5. XVII _____   8. XCI _____

3. XLVI _____   6. IV _____   9. M _____

III. Change the following fractions to the higher terms indicated:

1. $\dfrac{6}{7} = \dfrac{}{49}$ 3. $\dfrac{7}{10} = \dfrac{}{100}$ 5. $\dfrac{3}{8} = \dfrac{}{24}$

2. $\dfrac{3}{4} = \dfrac{}{16}$ 4. $\dfrac{1}{6} = \dfrac{}{36}$ 6. $\dfrac{4}{5} = \dfrac{}{20}$

IV. Reduce the following fractions to their lowest terms:

1. $\dfrac{8}{10}$ = _____   3. $\dfrac{5}{20}$ = _____   5. $\dfrac{4}{10}$ = _____

2. $\dfrac{2}{100}$ = _____   4. $\dfrac{6}{8}$ = _____   6. $\dfrac{5}{25}$ = _____

V. Change to whole or mixed numbers:

1. $\dfrac{28}{4}$ =   4. $\dfrac{35}{2}$ =   7. $\dfrac{69}{6}$ =

2. $\dfrac{19}{3}$ =   5. $\dfrac{77}{8}$ =   8. $\dfrac{136}{5}$ =

3. $\dfrac{12}{6}$ =   6. $\dfrac{88}{7}$ =   9. $\dfrac{230}{12}$ =

VI. Change the following mixed numbers to improper fractions:

1. $3\dfrac{3}{4}$ = _____   3. $16\dfrac{7}{8}$ = _____

2. $2\dfrac{1}{2}$ = _____   4. $25\dfrac{1}{5}$ = _____

VII. Circle the smaller fraction:

1. $\dfrac{3}{4}$ or $\dfrac{7}{8}$ 3. $\dfrac{2}{5}$ or $\dfrac{3}{10}$

2. $\dfrac{5}{6}$ or $\dfrac{9}{20}$ 4. $\dfrac{8}{9}$ or $\dfrac{6}{7}$

VIII. Add the following fractions:

1. $\dfrac{1}{4}$ 2. $2\dfrac{3}{5}$ 3. $\dfrac{1}{10}$ 4. $\dfrac{7}{9}$

$\dfrac{3}{8}$ $1\dfrac{1}{3}$ $\dfrac{3}{5}$ $\dfrac{9}{10}$

$\dfrac{2}{3}$ $4\dfrac{1}{2}$ $\dfrac{5}{8}$ $\dfrac{2}{15}$

IX. Subtract the following fractions and mixed numbers:

1. $\dfrac{4}{5} - \dfrac{1}{10}$ =   2. $2\dfrac{1}{4} - \dfrac{3}{8}$ =

3. $1\frac{6}{10} - \frac{3}{5} =$ 4. $8\frac{1}{2} - \frac{6}{8} =$

X. Multiply the following fractions and mixed numbers:

1. $\frac{2}{3} \times \frac{3}{8} =$ 3. $2\frac{1}{3} \times 15 =$

2. $15 \times 1\frac{4}{5} =$ 4. $6\frac{1}{2} \times 2 =$

XI. Write the words for the following decimals:

1. 1.6 _____

2. 20.75 _____

3. 200.04 _____

4. 450.251 _____

XII. Change the following fractions to decimals:

1. $\frac{4}{5} =$ _____   3. $\frac{6}{10} =$ _____

2. $\frac{3}{4} =$ _____   4. $\frac{1}{150} =$ _____

XIII. Change the following decimals to fractions:

1. $0.01 =$ _____   3. $0.4 =$ _____

2. $0.25 =$ _____   4. $0.005 =$ _____

XIV. Add the following decimals:

1. 0.059	2. 0.375	3. 0.6
0.61	0.5	0.4758
0.02	0.69	0.352

XV. Add the following decimals:

1. 256.789	2. 3.542	3. 45.65
83.45	89.65	915.78
66.5	33.3	1100.86

XVI. Subtract the following decimals:

1.   15.65
  −   8.35

2.   239.56
  − 131.02

3.   34.5
  − 26.5

4.   189
  −   5.29

XVII. Multiply the following decimals:

1.   622.4
  × 0.45

2.   150
  × 0.34

3. 910.24
  × 0.8

4.   88.40
  × 0.30

XVIII. Divide the following fractions and mixed numbers:

1. $\dfrac{5}{8} \div \dfrac{7}{10} =$

2. $2 \div \dfrac{3}{4} =$

3. $\dfrac{2}{9} \div 2\dfrac{1}{4} =$

4. $6\dfrac{1}{2} \div 3\dfrac{1}{2} =$

XIX. Divide the following numbers (round to thousandths, if necessary):

1. $86 \div 23.5$

2. $15.75 \div 2.5$

3. $156.8 \div 4.5$

4. $542.4 \div 45.2$

XX. Circle the smaller decimal:

1. 0.5 or 0.4

2. 0.75 or 0.078

3. 0.15 or 0.02

4. 0.25 or 0.35

XXI. Change the following fractions and mixed numbers to decimals:

1. $\dfrac{2}{5} =$

2. $\dfrac{7}{10} =$

3. $1\dfrac{4}{5} =$

4. $4\dfrac{1}{8} =$

XXII. Rewrite the following fractions as ratios, percentages, and decimals:

	Fraction	Ratio	Percentage	Decimal
1.	$\dfrac{6}{100}$ =	_____ =	_____ =	_____
2.	$\dfrac{3}{4}$ =	_____ =	_____ =	_____

	Fraction	Ratio	Percentage	Decimal
3.	$\dfrac{5}{1000}$ =	_____ =	_____ =	_____
4.	$\dfrac{1}{2}$ =	_____ =	_____ =	_____

XXIII. Solve the following percentages:

1. 4% of 60

2. 0.5% of 400

3. 0.4% of 800

4. 12% of 100

XXIV. Solve for x in the following proportions:

1. $1:6 = 7:x$

2. $5:16 = x:64$

3. $0.075:15 = 0.5:x$

4. $\dfrac{1}{10}:x = \dfrac{1}{4}:15$

1 ROMAN AND ARABIC NUMERALS

The nurse needs to know both Roman numerals and Arabic numbers for interpretation of drug orders and dosages. Roman numerals are used when the dosage of a drug is ordered in the apothecaries' system of measurement. Roman numerals above thirty are seldom used in prescribing dosage. When the small letter i is used for the Roman numeral one, it is usually dotted. When two or three ones are used, the last one may be written as a j. This is the only time that the letter j is used. The use of Arabic numbers has largely replaced the use of Roman numerals. This simplifies arithmetical processes. The following list shows the Arabic equivalents for Roman numerals.

Arabic	Roman	Arabic	Roman
1	I	19	XIX
2	II	20	XX
3	III	21	XXI
4	IV	22	XXII
5	V	23	XXIII
6	VI	24	XXIV
7	VII	25	XXV
8	VIII	26	XXVI
9	IX	27	XXVII
10	X	28	XXVIII
11	XI	29	XXIX
12	XII	30	XXX
13	XIII	40·	XL
14	XIV	50	L
15	XV	100	C
16	XVI	500	D
17	XVII	1000	M
18	XVIII		

A combination of Roman numerals can be used to express a numerical value, as shown in the preceding list. Basic Roman numerals include I, V,

X, L, C, D, and M. The following rules may be used to add or subtract value from the basic Roman numeral.

Rule for addition. *Placing one or more Roman numerals after the basic numeral adds to its value.* Beginning with a numeral, such as X (10), the same numeral or one of lesser value may be used to add value to the numeral.

EXAMPLES: XI = 11   XVI = 16

The numerals X, I, and C are not repeated more than three times. If that seems necessary, the rule for subtraction is used. The numerals V (5) and L (50) are not repeated successively to add value, but a numeral of higher value is used. For example, X is used to represent 10, rather than VV; and C is used to represent 100, rather than LL.

Rule for subtraction. *Placing one lower Roman numeral in front of the basic numeral removes value from it.*

EXAMPLES: IV = 4   IX = 9   XCI = 91

Exercise

Fill in the correct Roman numerals:

1. 8 _____	10. 30 _____	18. 1000 _____
2. 10 _____	11. 6 _____	19. 48 _____
3. 15 _____	12. 90 _____	20. 3 _____
4. 2 _____	13. 23 _____	21. 50 _____
5. 24 _____	14. 12 _____	22. 14 _____
6. 26 _____	15. 4 _____	23. 18 _____
7. 35 _____	16. 93 _____	24. 19 _____
8. 7 _____	17. 200 _____	25. 60 _____
9. 5 _____		

Fill in the correct Arabic numbers:

1. III _____	6. XXIX _____	11. XLVIII _____
2. XX _____	7. L _____	12. D _____
3. XXX _____	8. XIX _____	13. XVIII _____
4. XII _____	9. C _____	14. XV _____
5. XXIII _____	10. XL _____	15. X _____

16. VIII _____

17. XXXIX _____

18. IV _____

19. XXVIII _____

20. MM _____

21. VI _____

22. XXIV _____

23. XC _____

24. I _____

25. XVI _____

2 FRACTIONS

Proficiency in manipulating the addition, subtraction, multiplication, and division of both common fractions and decimals is necessary because the systems of weights and measures used to prescribe dosage often use common fractions or decimals for an amount less than one. Knowledge of and skill in converting a fraction to a decimal and vice versa enable the nurse to make necessary calculations when either decimals or fractions are used. The following review of fractions is designed to aid the student to recall basic knowledge of fractions.

A fraction is part of a whole number: ½, ¼, and so on. The number above the dividing line is called the *numerator.* It indicates the number of parts of the whole number that are being used; for example, ⅜ would mean that if something is divided into 8 parts, 3 of those 8 parts are being used. The number below the line is called the *denominator,* and it indicates the number of parts into which the whole is divided. Therefore, ⅜ means that the whole has been divided into 8 equal parts; ⅟₁₅₀ means that it has been divided into 150 equal parts and that 1 part of the 150 parts is being used. A fraction that has the same numerator and denominator equals the whole number 1. For example, 4/4 means that the whole number 1 has been divided into 4 equal parts, and all 4 parts of the fraction are being used.

In other words, *a denominator represents a divisor, a numerator represents a dividend, and, if division is performed, the answer obtained represents a quotient.*

Types of fractions may be defined as follows.

Common fractions. The numerator and denominator are both whole numbers.

EXAMPLES: $\dfrac{3}{4}$ $\dfrac{1}{2}$ $\dfrac{5}{2}$

Proper fractions (sometimes called "true fractions"). The numerator is always less than the denominator.

EXAMPLES: $\dfrac{5}{6}$ $\dfrac{1}{8}$ $\dfrac{1}{4}$

Improper fractions. The numerator is always larger than the denominator.

EXAMPLES: $\dfrac{4}{1}$ $\dfrac{6}{5}$ $\dfrac{16}{9}$

Improper fractions are changed to mixed numbers.
Mixed numbers. A whole number is combined with a fraction.

EXAMPLES: $2\dfrac{3}{4}$ $3\dfrac{1}{3}$ $2\dfrac{4}{5}$

Complex fractions. The numerator, the denominator, or both are a proper fraction, an improper fraction, or a mixed number.

EXAMPLES: $\dfrac{2}{1^1/_4}$ $\dfrac{^1/_2}{6}$ $\dfrac{^1/_3}{^1/_4}$

EXPRESSING FRACTIONS IN HIGHEST OR LOWEST TERMS

When both the numerator and the denominator of a fraction are multiplied by the same number, the value of the fraction remains unchanged.

EXAMPLES: $\dfrac{3}{4} \times \dfrac{2}{2} = \dfrac{6}{8} = \dfrac{3}{4}$ $\dfrac{5}{10} \times \dfrac{5}{5} = \dfrac{25}{50} = \dfrac{5}{10}$

A fraction may be reduced to lower terms by dividing both the numerator and the denominator by the same number. A fraction is said to have been reduced to its lowest terms when it is no longer possible to divide the numerator and denominator by the same number. Reducing a fraction to lowest terms does not change the value of the fraction.

Because it is easier to work with smaller fractions, it is usual to express fractions in their lowest terms—that is, to reduce them—by dividing both the numerator and the denominator by the same number.

EXAMPLES: $\dfrac{5}{10}\left(\div\dfrac{5}{5}\right) = \dfrac{1}{2}$ $\dfrac{3}{12}\left(\div\dfrac{3}{3}\right) = \dfrac{1}{4}$

It is also permissible to cancel out the larger figures.

EXAMPLES: $\dfrac{\overset{1}{\cancel{20}}}{\underset{5}{\cancel{100}}} = \dfrac{1}{5}$ $\dfrac{\overset{\overset{1}{\cancel{5}}}{\cancel{125}}}{\underset{\underset{2}{\cancel{10}}}{\cancel{250}}} = \dfrac{1}{2}$

14

Exercise

Express the following fractions in lowest terms:

1. $\dfrac{9}{48} =$

2. $\dfrac{6}{18} =$

3. $\dfrac{9}{12} =$

4. $\dfrac{6}{24} =$

5. $\dfrac{8}{32} =$

6. $\dfrac{125}{150} =$

7. $\dfrac{100}{200} =$

8. $\dfrac{6}{16} =$

9. $\dfrac{6}{9} =$

10. $\dfrac{8}{10} =$

11. $\dfrac{4}{12} =$

12. $\dfrac{8}{64} =$

13. $\dfrac{45}{90} =$

14. $\dfrac{7}{28} =$

15. $\dfrac{3}{12} =$

16. $\dfrac{4}{8} =$

17. $\dfrac{12}{144} =$

18. $\dfrac{25}{100} =$

19. $\dfrac{4}{20} =$

20. $\dfrac{36}{72} =$

21. $\dfrac{4}{10} =$

22. $\dfrac{14}{16} =$

23. $\dfrac{12}{20} =$

24. $\dfrac{6}{12} =$

25. $\dfrac{18}{72} =$

Exercise

Express the following fractions in the higher term, as indicated:

1. $\dfrac{6}{7} = \dfrac{}{49}$

2. $\dfrac{4}{5} = \dfrac{}{25}$

3. $\dfrac{1}{2} = \dfrac{}{10}$

4. $\dfrac{6}{11} = \dfrac{}{121}$

5. $\dfrac{2}{5} = \dfrac{}{10}$

6. $\dfrac{3}{8} = \dfrac{}{64}$

7. $\dfrac{2}{3} = \dfrac{}{21}$

8. $\dfrac{3}{10} = \dfrac{}{100}$

9. $\dfrac{2}{25} = \dfrac{}{50}$

10. $\dfrac{5}{8} = \dfrac{}{24}$

CHANGING IMPROPER FRACTIONS TO MIXED NUMBERS

An improper fraction can be changed to a mixed number by dividing the numerator by the denominator.

$$\text{EXAMPLE:} \quad \frac{6}{5} = 5\overline{)6.0}^{\,1.2} = 1\frac{2}{10} = 1\frac{1}{5} \left(\overset{1}{5\overline{)10}}\; \overset{}{\underset{5}{}} \right)$$

or

$$\frac{6}{5} = 6 \div 5 = 5\overline{)6.0}^{\,1.2}$$
$$\underline{5}$$
$$10$$
$$\underline{10}$$

Exercise

Change the following improper fractions to mixed or whole numbers, and reduce the answers to lowest terms:

1. $\dfrac{5}{3} =$

2. $\dfrac{10}{8} =$

3. $\dfrac{26}{12} =$

4. $\dfrac{24}{3} =$

5. $\dfrac{52}{3} =$

6. $\dfrac{51}{4} =$

7. $\dfrac{15}{2} =$

8. $\dfrac{75}{25} =$

9. $\dfrac{28}{9} =$

10. $\dfrac{50}{25} =$

11. $\dfrac{12}{4} =$

12. $\dfrac{11}{6} =$

13. $\dfrac{100}{10} =$

14. $\dfrac{14}{4} =$

15. $\dfrac{48}{12} =$

16. $\dfrac{36}{7} =$

17. $\dfrac{34}{4} =$

18. $\dfrac{42}{10} =$

19. $\dfrac{22}{5} =$

20. $\dfrac{42}{5} =$

21. $\dfrac{15}{10} =$

22. $\dfrac{24}{14} =$

23. $\dfrac{21}{9} =$

24. $\dfrac{3}{2} =$

25. $\dfrac{19}{3} =$

CHANGING MIXED NUMBERS TO IMPROPER FRACTIONS

A mixed number is changed to an improper fraction by multiplying the whole number by the denominator of the fraction and adding the numerator of the fraction to the result. Only a mixed number can be changed to an *improper* fraction, and the numerator will always be larger than the denominator.

EXAMPLES: $2\frac{1}{2} = \frac{(2 \times 2) + 1}{2} = \frac{5}{2}$ $3\frac{3}{4} = \frac{(3 \times 4) + 3}{4} = \frac{15}{4}$

Exercise

Change the following mixed numbers to improper fractions:

1. $7\frac{3}{4} =$

2. $18\frac{1}{2} =$

3. $9\frac{7}{10} =$

4. $50\frac{1}{2} =$

5. $6\frac{4}{5} =$

6. $3\frac{7}{8} =$

7. $2\frac{3}{7} =$

8. $4\frac{5}{8} =$

9. $3\frac{1}{2} =$

10. $5\frac{2}{3} =$

11. $16\frac{1}{4} =$

12. $2\frac{3}{5} =$

13. $6\frac{6}{100} =$

14. $4\frac{3}{4} =$

15. $6\frac{3}{5} =$

16. $8\frac{2}{50} =$

17. $10\frac{3}{4} =$

18. $3\frac{3}{8} =$

19. $20\frac{4}{9} =$

20. $7\frac{5}{8} =$

21. $4\frac{2}{5} =$

22. $7\frac{1}{8} =$

23. $9\frac{3}{5} =$

24. $2\frac{8}{27} =$

25. $21\frac{6}{7} =$

COMPARING THE SIZE OF FRACTIONS

It is sometimes necessary to determine which of two fractions is the larger, or, if more than two, which is the largest. Proceed as follows:

17

(a) *If all the numerators are 1, the larger the denominator, the smaller the fraction.* For example, $\frac{1}{150}$ is smaller than $\frac{1}{125}$. To demonstrate this point, divide a circle into eight equal parts.

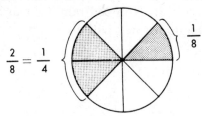

$$\frac{2}{8} = \frac{1}{4}$$

$$\frac{1}{8}$$

The size of the parts demonstrates that the fraction $\frac{1}{8}$ is smaller than $\frac{1}{4}$ ($\frac{2}{8}$), even though the whole number 8 is larger than the whole number 4.

Exercise

Circle the *larger* fraction in each of the following pairs:

1. $\frac{1}{200}$ or $\frac{1}{100}$

2. $\frac{1}{3}$ or $\frac{1}{5}$

3. $\frac{1}{12}$ or $\frac{1}{24}$

4. $\frac{1}{100}$ or $\frac{1}{150}$

5. $\frac{1}{175}$ or $\frac{1}{125}$

6. $\frac{1}{49}$ or $\frac{1}{72}$

7. $\frac{1}{6}$ or $\frac{1}{10}$

8. $\frac{1}{25}$ or $\frac{1}{75}$

9. $\frac{3}{250}$ or $\frac{3}{125}$

10. $\frac{4}{150}$ or $\frac{1}{150}$

11. $\frac{2}{11}$ or $\frac{2}{7}$

12. $\frac{6}{15}$ or $\frac{9}{15}$

(b) *If the fractions have the same denominator but different numerators (for example, $\frac{1}{8}$, $\frac{3}{8}$, $\frac{7}{8}$), the fraction with the largest numerator is the largest fraction, so $\frac{7}{8}$ would be the largest of these three fractions.*

Exercise

Circle the *smaller* fraction in each of the following pairs:

13. $\frac{16}{135}$ or $\frac{12}{135}$

14. $\frac{1}{10}$ or $\frac{9}{10}$

15. $\frac{1}{6}$ or $\frac{5}{6}$

16. $\frac{2}{25}$ or $\frac{4}{25}$

17. $\frac{1}{125}$ or $\frac{6}{125}$

18. $\frac{8}{130}$ or $\frac{12}{130}$

19. $\frac{7}{8}$ or $\frac{5}{8}$

20. $\frac{9}{80}$ or $\frac{11}{80}$

21. $\frac{3}{50}$ or $\frac{4}{50}$

22. $\frac{6}{7}$ or $\frac{5}{7}$

23. $\frac{1}{150}$ or $\frac{1}{100}$

24. $\frac{4}{10}$ or $\frac{6}{10}$

(c) *When all the numerators and denominators differ, as in $2/3$, $5/6$, $7/9$, it is possible to determine which is largest and which is smallest by changing all the fractions so that all the denominators are the same.* This is done by finding a denominator that is common to all the fractions. For the fractions, $2/3$, $5/6$, $7/9$, the number 18 could be the common denominator. Each of these denominators would divide into 18; that is, they could all have 18 as a dividend. Directions for finding the common denominator are given in Chapter 3. Both the *numerator* and the *denominator* of a fraction would have to be multiplied by the same number to keep the fractions balanced.

EXAMPLES: $\frac{2}{3} \times \frac{6}{6} = \frac{12}{18}$ $\frac{5}{6} \times \frac{3}{3} = \frac{15}{18}$ $\frac{7}{9} \times \frac{2}{2} = \frac{14}{18}$

It is seen that $15/18$ is the largest fraction, and $5/6$ would therefore be the largest fraction of the group.

Exercise

Circle the *larger* fraction in each of the following pairs:

25. $\frac{5}{6}$ or $\frac{8}{9}$

26. $\frac{4}{5}$ or $\frac{5}{6}$

27. $\frac{12}{25}$ or $\frac{5}{9}$

28. $\frac{3}{4}$ or $\frac{4}{5}$

29. $\frac{7}{9}$ or $\frac{5}{8}$

30. $\frac{9}{40}$ or $\frac{7}{30}$

31. $\frac{7}{30}$ or $\frac{4}{5}$

32. $\frac{7}{8}$ or $\frac{5}{9}$

33. $\frac{6}{50}$ or $\frac{4}{25}$

34. $\frac{3}{10}$ or $\frac{2}{9}$

35. $\frac{4}{150}$ or $\frac{3}{50}$

3 ADDING FRACTIONS

To add two or more fractions, it is necessary to find the common denominator. Several methods can be used. One method is to find the smallest denominator that is common to all the fractions to be added. In simple problems, this is likely to be the largest denominator in a series of fractions. In more complex problems, *it may be necessary to multiply denominators to find a common denominator.*

After placing the fractions in a column for addition, find the common denominator. In the following example, the common denominator is represented by 20, the largest denominator of the fractions:

EXAMPLE: Add $\dfrac{1}{2}, \dfrac{1}{5}, \dfrac{1}{10}, \dfrac{1}{20}$

The fractions are then changed as indicated to obtain fractions of equal value, each with the same denominator. This is done by dividing the new denominator by the original denominator and multiplying the result by the numerator of the original fraction to obtain the new numerator. Next, the numerators of the fractions are added together and placed over the common denominator. Then the fraction that is obtained as the answer is reduced to lowest terms.

Two methods are used to illustrate addition of fractions. In both methods demonstrated, the fractions are placed directly beneath each other. Next, the original fractions are changed to new fractions of equal value, each with the same denominator. In the method on the left, the total equivalent fractions are listed. In the method on the right, the numerators of the fractions are listed separately from the common denominator for ease in addition. In both methods, the numerators are added and placed over the common denominator.

EXAMPLE A: Add $\dfrac{1}{2}, \dfrac{1}{5}, \dfrac{1}{10}, \dfrac{1}{20}$

$$\frac{1}{2} = \frac{10}{20} \qquad \text{or} \qquad \left.\begin{array}{c}\frac{1}{2} \\ \frac{1}{5} \\ \frac{1}{10} \\ \frac{1}{20}\end{array}\right] \overline{\begin{array}{c}20 \\ 10 \\ 4 \\ 2 \\ 1\end{array}} \quad \begin{array}{c}\left(\frac{10}{20}\right) \\ \left(\frac{4}{20}\right) \\ \left(\frac{2}{20}\right) \\ \left(\frac{1}{20}\right)\end{array}$$

$$\frac{1}{5} = \frac{4}{20}$$

$$\frac{1}{10} = \frac{2}{20}$$

$$\frac{1}{20} = \frac{1}{20}$$

$$\frac{17}{20} \qquad\qquad \frac{17}{20}\bigg|\frac{17}{20}$$

When adding mixed numbers, the whole numbers are placed directly underneath each other, as are the fractions.

EXAMPLE B: Add $1\frac{1}{2}$, $2\frac{2}{3}$, $3\frac{3}{4}$

$$1\frac{1}{2} = 1\frac{6}{12} \qquad \text{or} \qquad \left.\begin{array}{c}1\frac{1}{2} \\[4pt] 2\frac{2}{3} \\[4pt] 3\frac{3}{4}\end{array}\right] \overline{\begin{array}{c}12 \\ 6 \\ 8 \\ 9\end{array}}$$

$$2\frac{2}{3} = 2\frac{8}{12}$$

$$3\frac{3}{4} = 3\frac{9}{12}$$

$$6\frac{23}{12} = 7\frac{11}{12} \qquad\qquad 6\bigg|\frac{23}{12} = 1\frac{11}{12}$$

$$+\ 1\frac{11}{12}$$

$$7\frac{11}{12}$$

When adding mixed numbers, the fractions are added first, and then the whole numbers. If addition of the fractions yields an improper fraction, it is changed to a mixed number, and the whole number obtained is added to the other whole numbers.

Exercise

Add the following fractions and mixed numbers, and reduce the answers to lowest terms:

1. $\dfrac{4}{5}$
   $\dfrac{9}{30}$
   $\dfrac{5}{90}$

2. $\dfrac{9}{72}$
   $\dfrac{7}{8}$
   $\dfrac{4}{9}$

3. $\dfrac{3}{4}$

      $\dfrac{7}{16}$

      $\dfrac{5}{8}$

      $\dfrac{1}{32}$

7. $22\dfrac{1}{6}$

    $15\dfrac{4}{9}$

    $36\dfrac{2}{27}$

4. $\dfrac{1}{2}$

      $\dfrac{3}{20}$

      $\dfrac{7}{10}$

      $\dfrac{9}{40}$

8. $\dfrac{1}{9}$

      $\dfrac{3}{27}$

      $\dfrac{4}{18}$

      $\dfrac{2}{3}$

5. $\dfrac{3}{4}$

      $\dfrac{11}{32}$

      $\dfrac{7}{8}$

      $\dfrac{5}{16}$

9. $\dfrac{5}{32}$

      $\dfrac{1}{48}$

      $\dfrac{1}{24}$

      $\dfrac{1}{16}$

6. $7\dfrac{5}{6}$

    $\dfrac{8}{9}$

    $\dfrac{7}{8}$

    $\dfrac{1}{6}$

10. $43\dfrac{1}{2}$

    $78\dfrac{1}{8}$

    $10\dfrac{4}{5}$

11. $\dfrac{3}{4}$

    $\dfrac{5}{6}$

    $\dfrac{1}{8}$

    $\dfrac{2}{32}$

16. $1\dfrac{2}{3}$

    $3\dfrac{5}{8}$

    $2\dfrac{1}{6}$

12. $20\dfrac{3}{4}$

    $14\dfrac{1}{2}$

    $16\dfrac{1}{4}$

17. $18\dfrac{3}{8}$

    $12\dfrac{3}{4}$

    $16\dfrac{1}{6}$

13. $5\dfrac{2}{3}$

    $1\dfrac{5}{8}$

    $6\dfrac{3}{4}$

18. $4\dfrac{1}{8}$

    $\dfrac{2}{3}$

    $12\dfrac{3}{4}$

14. $\dfrac{4}{21}$

    $6\dfrac{3}{7}$

    $\dfrac{1}{84}$

19. $\dfrac{6}{8}$

    $\dfrac{1}{4}$

    $3\dfrac{1}{10}$

15. $9\dfrac{7}{32}$

    $\dfrac{3}{16}$

    $7\dfrac{1}{48}$

20. $52\dfrac{1}{12}$

    $3\dfrac{2}{3}$

    $4\dfrac{3}{4}$

4 SUBTRACTING FRACTIONS

In subtracting fractions, as in adding fractions, it is necessary to find the common denominator. In the examples given, method **(A)** shows the total equivalent fractions and method **(B)** lists the common denominator separate from the numerators of the fractions.

EXAMPLE: $\dfrac{3}{4} - \dfrac{1}{2}$

(A)

$$\dfrac{3}{4} = \dfrac{3}{4}$$
$$-\dfrac{1}{2} = -\dfrac{2}{4}$$
$$\overline{\dfrac{1}{4}}$$

or

(B) 4— Common denominator

$$\begin{array}{r} \dfrac{3}{4} \\ -\dfrac{1}{2} \end{array} \begin{array}{|l} 3 \\ 2 \end{array}$$ Numerators

$$\dfrac{1}{4} \Big| 1$$

If the fraction to be subtracted is larger than that from which it is to be subtracted, a whole number (1) must be borrowed from the whole number in the mixed number and then added to the fraction.

EXAMPLE: $2\dfrac{1}{4} - 1\dfrac{1}{2}$

(A)

$$2\dfrac{1}{4} \qquad 2\dfrac{1}{4} = 1\dfrac{5}{4}$$
$$-1\dfrac{1}{2} = -1\dfrac{2}{4} = -1\dfrac{2}{4}$$
$$\overline{\dfrac{3}{4}}$$

or

(B)

$$2\dfrac{1}{4} \begin{array}{|l} \overset{1}{}\overset{4}{} \\ 1 \ \left(\text{plus } \dfrac{4}{4}, \text{ or } 1\right) = \dfrac{5}{4} \end{array}$$
$$-1\dfrac{1}{2} \begin{array}{|l} 2 \ (\text{one half of 4}) = -\dfrac{2}{4} \end{array}$$
$$\dfrac{3}{4} \Big| \dfrac{3}{4} \qquad\qquad\qquad \dfrac{3}{4}$$

24

Exercise

Subtract the following fractions and mixed numbers, and reduce the answers to lowest terms:

1. $\dfrac{3}{20}$

   $-\dfrac{1}{10}$

2. $\dfrac{4}{27}$

   $-\dfrac{1}{9}$

3. $\dfrac{3}{5}$

   $-\dfrac{4}{10}$

4. $\dfrac{5}{8}$

   $-\dfrac{3}{16}$

5. $\dfrac{8}{10}$

   $-\dfrac{4}{5}$

6. $\dfrac{9}{10}$

   $-\dfrac{3}{5}$

7. $\dfrac{10}{16}$

   $-\dfrac{3}{8}$

8. $2\dfrac{4}{5}$

   $-\dfrac{7}{10}$

9. $14\dfrac{4}{5}$

   $-7\dfrac{9}{30}$

10. $1\dfrac{1}{12}$

    $-\dfrac{3}{24}$

11. $2\dfrac{1}{4}$

    $-1\dfrac{1}{2}$

12. $6\dfrac{3}{8}$

    $-2\dfrac{1}{4}$

13. $12\frac{3}{5}$

$-\ 2\frac{1}{5}$

14. $16\frac{1}{3}$

$-\ 3\frac{2}{3}$

15. $185\frac{1}{24}$

$-\ 16\frac{5}{12}$

16. $25\frac{1}{2}$

$-\ 15\frac{1}{4}$

17. $63\frac{2}{3}$

$-\ 5\frac{1}{15}$

18. $28\frac{3}{4}$

$-\ 18\frac{2}{6}$

19. $45\frac{1}{4}$

$-\ 16\frac{3}{4}$

20. $65\frac{1}{6}$

$-\ 18\frac{1}{12}$

21. $87\frac{3}{5}$

$-\ 42\frac{7}{10}$

22. $180\frac{6}{7}$

$-\ 23\frac{3}{14}$

23. $195\frac{1}{12}$

$-\ 140\frac{3}{5}$

24. $134\frac{3}{25}$

$-\ 39\frac{3}{50}$

25. $48\frac{3}{5}$

$-\ 10\frac{1}{10}$

5 MULTIPLYING FRACTIONS

To multiply a fraction by a whole number, multiply the numerator by the whole number and place this answer over the denominator, which remains unchanged.

EXAMPLE: $3 \times \dfrac{2}{3} = \dfrac{6}{3} = 2$

If desired, the whole number can be changed to an improper fraction by placing the whole number over a denominator of 1. In this case, the numerators are then multiplied together, as are the denominators.

EXAMPLE: $3 \times \dfrac{2}{3} = \dfrac{3}{1} \times \dfrac{2}{3} = \dfrac{6}{3} = 2$

Cancellation can be carried out by dividing a numerator and a denominator by the same number.

EXAMPLE: $3 \times \dfrac{2}{3} = \dfrac{\overset{1}{\cancel{3}}}{1} \times \dfrac{2}{\underset{1}{\cancel{3}}} = 2$

To multiply fractions, multiply all the numerators together and place this answer (the product) over the product of all the denominators. Again, cancellation may be carried out.

EXAMPLE: $\dfrac{1}{2} \times \dfrac{2}{3} = \dfrac{2}{6} = \dfrac{1}{3}$ or $\dfrac{1}{\underset{1}{\cancel{2}}} \times \dfrac{\overset{1}{\cancel{2}}}{3} = \dfrac{1}{3}$

NOTE: In fractions the × (multiplication sign) also means "of," so ½ of ⅔ means ½ × ⅔.

To multiply mixed numbers, change the whole number and fraction to an *improper fraction*. Then multiply all the numerators together and place this product over the product of the denominators. Cancellation may be used in solving the problem.

EXAMPLE: $2\frac{1}{2} \times 3\frac{1}{8} = \frac{5}{2} \times \frac{25}{8} = \frac{125}{16} = 7\frac{13}{16}$

Exercise

Multiply the following fractions and mixed numbers, and reduce the answers to lowest terms:

1. $\frac{1}{2} \times \frac{7}{8} =$

2. $\frac{6}{7} \times \frac{14}{33} =$

3. $\frac{3}{8} \times \frac{8}{9} =$

4. $\frac{3}{5} \times \frac{5}{12} =$

5. $\frac{4}{9} \times \frac{9}{10} =$

6. $\frac{1}{5} \times \frac{5}{6} =$

7. $\frac{1}{8} \times \frac{5}{6} =$

8. $\frac{1}{3} \times \frac{6}{12} =$

9. $\frac{8}{9} \times \frac{5}{6} =$

10. $\frac{4}{9} \times \frac{4}{5} =$

11. $\frac{1}{16} \times \frac{3}{5} =$

12. $\frac{2}{25} \times \frac{7}{20} =$

13. $\frac{2}{3} \times \frac{9}{25} =$

14. $2\frac{11}{12} \times 1\frac{5}{8} =$

15. $5\frac{1}{4} \times 2\frac{5}{6} =$

16. $1\frac{7}{8} \times 3\frac{1}{4} =$

17. $6\frac{1}{2} \times 4\frac{5}{8} =$

18. $8\frac{1}{5} \times 8\frac{4}{5} =$

19. $6\frac{2}{3} \times 1\frac{1}{12} =$

20. $8\frac{1}{4} \times 4\frac{4}{5} \times 2\frac{1}{2} =$

21. $3\frac{1}{2} \times 6\frac{1}{4} \times 8\frac{1}{8} =$

22. $9\frac{3}{4} \times 8\frac{2}{3} \times 2\frac{1}{12} =$

23. $11\frac{1}{2} \times 8\frac{6}{7} \times \frac{3}{56} =$

24. $20\frac{1}{4} \times 22\frac{1}{3} \times 10\frac{1}{2} =$

25. $18\frac{1}{2} \times 10\frac{1}{3} \times 4\frac{1}{4} =$

6 DIVIDING FRACTIONS

To divide a whole number by a fraction, invert the fraction and multiply.

EXAMPLE: Divide 6 by $\frac{2}{3}$ $6 \div \frac{2}{3} = 6 \times \frac{3}{2} = \frac{18}{2} = 9$

Cancellation may be carried out if the whole number is changed to an improper fraction by placing the whole number over the denominator 1.

EXAMPLE: $6 \div \frac{2}{3} = \frac{\cancel{6}^{3}}{1} \times \frac{3}{\cancel{2}_{1}} = 9$

To divide one fraction by another, invert the fraction that is the divisor, that is, the second fraction, and multiply. Again, cancellation may be used.

EXAMPLE: Divide $\frac{4}{5}$ by $\frac{1}{5}$

$$\frac{4}{5} \div \frac{1}{5} = \frac{4}{\cancel{5}_{1}} \times \frac{\cancel{5}^{1}}{1} = 4$$

To divide mixed numbers, first change the mixed numbers to improper fractions, invert the divisor—that is, the second fraction—and then multiply.

EXAMPLE: Divide $2\frac{1}{2}$ by $3\frac{1}{8}$ $\frac{5}{2} \div \frac{25}{8} = \frac{\cancel{5}^{1}}{\cancel{2}_{1}} \times \frac{\cancel{8}^{4}}{\cancel{25}_{5}} = \frac{4}{5}$

When the numerator, the denominator, or both are fractions or mixed numbers, such as $\frac{1^{3}/_{4}}{^{5}/_{6}}$ *or* $\frac{3^{1}/_{2}}{2}$, *it is necessary first to clear the mixed numbers*

29

and then *to divide the numerator by the denominator* because the line separating the numerator and the denominator means the numerator is to be divided by the denominator. Consider the fraction $\dfrac{1^3/_4}{5/_6}$. This fraction would become $\dfrac{7/_4}{5/_6}$ after clearing the 1¾ in the numerator. This would mean ⁷⁄₄ ÷ ⁵⁄₆, which becomes ⁷⁄₄ × ⁶⁄₅ (inverting the divisor), resulting in the fraction ⁴²⁄₂₀, which equals 2²⁄₂₀. Reducing ²⁄₂₀ to its lowest terms by dividing both terms of the fraction by 2 shows the answer to be 2¹⁄₁₀.

Exercise

Divide the following fractions and mixed numbers, and reduce the answers to lowest terms:

1. $\dfrac{2}{6} \div \dfrac{3}{12} =$

2. $\dfrac{3}{8} \div \dfrac{5}{6} =$

3. $\dfrac{1}{100} \div \dfrac{7}{10} =$

4. $\dfrac{3}{20} \div \dfrac{2}{5} =$

5. $\dfrac{1}{12} \div \dfrac{3}{24} =$

6. $\dfrac{1}{25} \div \dfrac{3}{50} =$

7. $\dfrac{5}{8} \div \dfrac{5}{16} =$

8. $\dfrac{3}{4} \div \dfrac{9}{5} =$

9. $\dfrac{2}{25} \div \dfrac{7}{75} =$

10. $1\dfrac{2}{3} \div 6\dfrac{1}{5} =$

11. $1\dfrac{1}{2} \div \dfrac{3}{4} =$

12. $\dfrac{1}{150} \div \dfrac{1}{200} =$

13. $12\dfrac{3}{5} \div 8\dfrac{1}{2} =$

14. $\dfrac{7}{8} \div 2\dfrac{4}{5} =$

15. $\dfrac{1}{75} \div \dfrac{1}{25} =$

16. $\dfrac{1}{60} \div \dfrac{1}{2} =$

17. $2\dfrac{2}{3} \div \dfrac{1}{2} =$

18. $7\dfrac{3}{4} \div \dfrac{1}{150} =$

19. $6\dfrac{3}{5} \div \dfrac{7}{10} =$

20. $14\dfrac{1}{3} \div 3\dfrac{7}{8} =$

21. $3\dfrac{7}{8} \div \dfrac{3}{40} =$

22. $240 \div 3\dfrac{1}{2} =$

23. $17\dfrac{3}{4} \div 8\dfrac{1}{8} =$ 25. $45\dfrac{1}{4} \div 18\dfrac{1}{2} =$

24. $50 \div 12\dfrac{1}{2} =$

7 DECIMALS

When working with decimals, it is essential to know that *all figures to the left of the decimal point are whole numbers, and those to the right are decimal fractions,* representing a part of one whole. Decimals are read as follows:

.5   6   2

Tenths   Hundredths   Thousandths

Tenths are directly after the decimal point; hundredths are two places after the decimal point; thousandths are three places after the decimal point. A fourth figure would be ten thousandths, a fifth would be hundred thousandths, and so on. The above figure would be read five hundred sixty-two thousandths. Since numbers placed in front of the decimal point are read as whole numbers, 2.562 would be read two and five hundred sixty-two thousandths.

Exercise

Write the words for the following decimals:

1. 8.35 _____

2. 0.06 _____

3. 23.7 _____

4. 1.23 _____

5. 3.821 _____

6. 0.9 _____

7. 0.8 _____

8. 0.009 _____

9. 2.5 _____

10. 4.06 _____

11. 0.01 _____

12. 0.015 _____

Fractions may be changed to their decimal forms by dividing the numerator by the denominator.

EXAMPLES: $\dfrac{3}{5} = 3 \div 5 = 0.6$ $\dfrac{7}{8} = 8\overline{)7.000}$ $\begin{array}{r} 0.875 \\ \hline \end{array}$

$$\begin{array}{r} 6\ 4 \\ \hline 60 \\ 56 \\ \hline 40 \\ 40 \\ \hline \end{array}$$

or

$\dfrac{3}{5} = \dfrac{5\overline{)3.0}}{0.6}$

Exercise

Change the following fractions to decimals, rounding to thousandths:

1. $\dfrac{1}{25}$ _____

2. $\dfrac{3}{50}$ _____

3. $\dfrac{5}{8}$ _____

4. $\dfrac{2}{5}$ _____

5. $\dfrac{3}{150}$ _____

6. $\dfrac{3}{4}$ _____

7. $\dfrac{1}{2}$ _____

8. $\dfrac{1}{10}$ _____

9. $\dfrac{6}{7}$ _____

10. $\dfrac{2}{25}$ _____

11. $\dfrac{3}{8}$ _____

12. $\dfrac{3}{25}$ _____

13. $\dfrac{9}{10}$ _____

14. $\dfrac{5}{9}$ _____

15. $\dfrac{4}{5}$ _____

16. $\dfrac{6}{10}$ _____

17. $\frac{1}{50}$ _____

18. $\frac{7}{1000}$ _____

19. $\frac{5}{12}$ _____

20. $\frac{3}{4}$ _____

21. $\frac{3}{800}$ _____

22. $\frac{1}{200}$ _____

23. $\frac{7}{10}$ _____

24. $\frac{5}{6}$ _____

25. $\frac{1}{5}$ _____

Decimals may be changed to fractions by dropping the decimal point and using the proper denominator: 0.5 becomes ⁵⁄₁₀ or ½ (expressing the fraction in its lowest terms). Similarly, 0.75 becomes ⁷⁵⁄₁₀₀ (because the decimal is read seventy-five one hundredths); and 0.005 becomes ⁵⁄₁₀₀₀. The fraction ⁷⁵⁄₁₀₀ expressed in its lowest terms becomes ¾, and ⁵⁄₁₀₀₀ becomes ¹⁄₂₀₀.

The same principle applies when a decimal containing a whole number is to be changed to a mixed number. Thus, 1.5 becomes 1⁵⁄₁₀ or is reduced to its lowest terms, 1½.

Exercise

Change the following decimals to fractions, and reduce the answers to lowest terms:

1. 0.5 _____

2. 0.72 _____

3. 0.40 _____

4. 0.065 _____

5. 0.85 _____

6. 0.12 _____

7. 1.5 _____

8. 0.375 _____

9. 0.06 _____

10. 0.20 _____

11. 0.001 _____

12. 0.04 _____

13. 0.65 _____

14. 0.0006 _____

15. 0.6 _____

16. 0.28 _____

17. 0.0005 _____

18. 0.1 _____

19. 2.8 _____

20. 0.75 _____

21. 0.25 _____

22. 0.00004 _____

23. 0.9 _____

24. 0.15 _____

25. 5.2 _____

8 ADDING DECIMALS

When adding decimals, place the figures in columns, with the decimal points exactly underneath each other. Aligning the decimal points and digits in columns helps to avoid errors in addition.

Zeros may be added after the decimal number without changing its value. The empty space following a decimal number is the same as a zero.

EXAMPLE: Add 0.9, 0.65, 0.225, 0.86

```
0.900
0.650
0.225
0.860
2.635
```

A whole number in a decimal is placed to the left of the decimal point, as mentioned previously. Zeros preceding a whole number do not change its value. Thus, 0002.6 is the same as 2.6.

Exercise

Add the following decimals:

1. 4.8, 5.3, 9.6

2. 0.003, 2.5, 60.8, 3

3. 5.4, 8.2, 16.8

4. 20.3, 18.35, 20.65

5. 0.005, 1.05, 6.25

6. 10.2, 13.5, 16.8

7. 4.29, 1.001, 0.023

8. 9.63, 0.25, 1.395

9. 42.006, 3.7, 2.48

10. 9.5, 8.752, 4.25

11. 54.7, 0.227, 0.238

12. 9.7, 2.063, 14.695

13. 8.25, 6.50, 18.005

14. 8.75, 4.4, 300.276

15. 82.327, 4.05, 1.1

16. 0.2, 0.06, 0.005

17. 36.2, 0.641, 29

18. 7.24, 84.6, 0.003

19. 3.006, 5.203, 7.4

20. 29.1, 0.0001, 0.010

21. 6.857, 921.2, 7.21

22. 87.5, 4.237, 210.01

23. 14.77, 18.2, 0.004

24. 56.6, 8.021, 0.03

25. 8.777, 43.5, 122.66

9 SUBTRACTING DECIMALS

When subtracting decimals, observe the same rule as for adding decimals: the columns of digits are aligned so that *the decimal points are placed directly underneath each other.* Otherwise, subtracting decimals is the same as subtracting whole numbers.

EXAMPLE: Subtract 3.22 from 9.54

$$
\begin{array}{r}
9.54 \\
- \ 3.22 \\
\hline
6.32
\end{array}
$$

Exercise

Subtract the following decimals:

1. 6.91 − 3.78

2. 5.798 − 2.514

3. 2.6 − 1.3

4. 65.3 − 20.2

5. 49.27 − 31.06

6. 26.8 − 0.05

7. 17.5 − 14.2

8. 7.52 − 4.8

9. 15.02 − 11.91

10. 4.7 − 1.825

11. 107.5 − 73.7

12. 35.2 − 17.56

13. 114.3 − 86.8

14. 8.16 − 3.04

15. 195.6 − 179.73

16. 44.37 − 29.17

17. 4.76 − 0.87

18. 97.2 − 6.004

19. 203.5 − 73.79

20. 125.325 − 37.02

21. 85.7 − 4.92

22. 9.5 − 6.37

23. 1.2 − 0.8

24. 37.5 − 29.67

25. 342.21 − 88.792

10 MULTIPLYING DECIMALS

When multiplying decimals, first align the digits on the far right of the numbers to be multiplied, then multiply disregarding the decimal points, and finally place the decimal point in the product by counting from the right the number of places equal to the total number of decimal places in both the multiplier (number by which another is to be multiplied) and the multiplicand (number multiplied).

EXAMPLES:

$$
\begin{array}{r}
3562 \\
\times\ .65 \\
\hline
178\ 10 \\
2137\ 2 \\
\hline
2315.30
\end{array}
\qquad
\begin{array}{r}
3.56 \\
\times\ .25 \\
\hline
1780 \\
712 \\
\hline
0.8900
\end{array}
$$

In the first example, there are two decimal places in the multiplier, and there is no decimal in the multiplicand; therefore, mark off two decimal places from the right in the product. In the second example, there are two decimal places in the multiplicand and in the multiplier; therefore, mark off four decimal places in the product.

The number of digits to the right of the decimal point in the product obtained equals the sum of the number of digits to the right of the decimals in the multiplier and multiplicand.

Zeros may be removed from the end of the decimal number without changing its value. This simplifies multiplication.

EXAMPLE: 7.23Ø × 6.4ØØ

$$
\begin{array}{r}
7.23 \\
\times\ 6.4 \\
\hline
2892 \\
4338 \\
\hline
46.272
\end{array}
$$

There is sometimes confusion in multiplying two figures if a zero is contained in one or both of them.

EXAMPLES:

207	225	360
× 55	× 304	× 150
1035	900	18000
1035	6750	360
11385	68400	54000

The first example illustrates that multiplication of a zero by another number results in zero. The second example illustrates that multiplication of a number by a zero results in zero. The third example illustrates that multiplication of a zero by a zero results in zero.

When multiplying by tenths, hundredths, or thousandths, it is quicker to move the decimal point one, two, or three places, respectively, to the right. When multiplying a figure by 10, move the decimal point one place to the right, since that is the position for tenths.

EXAMPLE: $56 \times 10 = 560$ (56ₓ0.)

It is understood that there is a decimal point after any whole number. The figure 56 becomes 56. by placing a decimal point after it. To multiply 56 by 10, move the decimal point one place to the right.

When multiplying a figure by 100, move the decimal point two places to the right, which is the position for hundredths.

EXAMPLES: $85 \times 100 = 8500$ $1.7 \times 100 = 1{_x}70.$

When multiplying a figure by 1000, move the decimal point three places to the right, since that is the position for thousandths.

EXAMPLES: $76 \times 1000 = 76{,}000$ $0.75 \times 1000 = {_x}750.\cancel{0}\cancel{0}$

Exercise

Multiply the following decimals:

1. 0.7×8

2. 4.5×3

3. 15.5×0.05

4. 1.50×8.7

5. 24.5×13

6. 9.16×7

7. 27.537×1.08

8. 40.2×7.53

9. 7.4×82.91

10. 0.643×0.002

11. 0.7 × 88

12. 0.75 × 102.6

13. 37.2 × 8.95

14. 0.0062 × 7.4

15. 0.729 × 5

16. 0.27 × 0.02

17. 204.9 × 12

18. 4.0 × 80

19. 8.8 × 6.9

20. 4.6 × 7.19

21. 0.2 × 9.56

22. 0.4 × 10

23. 0.87 × 96.7

24. 45 × 0.3

25. 9.93 × 79.3

11 DIVIDING DECIMALS

Dividing decimals is slightly more complicated than adding, subtracting, or multiplying decimals. *If the divisor is a decimal, move the decimal point the required number of places to the right to make the decimal a whole number. It then becomes necessary to move the decimal point in the dividend the same number of places to avoid changing the value of the quotient. Place the decimal point in the quotient directly above the decimal point in the dividend.*

> EXAMPLE: Divide 0.325 by 0.64

$$
\begin{array}{r}
.507 \\
{}_x64.\overline{)}{}_x32.500 \\
32\ 0 \\
\hline
500 \\
\underline{448}
\end{array}
$$

Then proceed to divide as usual. Recheck the placement of the decimal point in the quotient, and recheck the arithmetic done.

When dividing a figure by 10, 100, or 1000, it is easier to move the decimal point one place, two places, or three places, respectively, to the left.

> EXAMPLES: $55 \div 10 = 5.5$ (5.5_x)
> $55 \div 100 = .55$ $(.55_x)$
> $55 \div 1000 = .055$ $(.055_x)$

Exercise

Divide the following decimals, rounding to thousandths:

1. $350 \div 2.5$

2. $74.4 \div 80$

3. $32.4 \div 12.5$

4. $0.2 \div 5$

5. 275 ÷ 0.05

6. 0.006 ÷ 0.05

7. 0.042 ÷ 3.3

8. 2 ÷ 0.5

9. 6.4 ÷ 0.5

10. 24.57 ÷ 2.7

11. 15 ÷ 7.5

12. 0.9 ÷ 0.6

13. 5.2 ÷ 2.02

14. 20.15 ÷ 5.01

15. 1 ÷ 0.1

16. 0.04 ÷ 26.1

17. 1.4 ÷ 70

18. 15.50 ÷ 3.6

19. 0.0798 ÷ 0.19

20. 9.72 ÷ 5.4

21. 0.67 ÷ .7

22. 1.5 ÷ 0.3

23. 7.2 ÷ 0.8

24. 4.01 ÷ 12

25. 306.8 ÷ 7.62

COMPARING THE VALUE OF DECIMALS

The value of a decimal remains unchanged when one or more zeros are appended to it. For example, 0.5 may be written as 0.50 without changing its value. One method of comparing the size of decimals is as follows: append zeros as necessary to equalize the number of decimal places in each decimal, and then compare the size of the resulting number.

EXAMPLE: Which of the following decimals is larger, 0.5 or 0.085?

0.5 = 0.500 (add zeros to get the same number of decimal places for each fraction)

It will be seen that 0.500 is larger than 0.085.

Exercise

Circle the *larger* decimal in the following pairs of decimals:

1. 0.06 or 0.6

2. 0.12 or 0.1

3. 0.9 or 0.09

4. 2.48 or 0.5

5. 0.840 or 0.084

6. 0.850 or 0.76

7. 0.2 or 0.02

8. 0.46 or 0.725

9. 0.87 or 0.9

10. 0.0256 or 0.04

11. 0.06 or 0.015

12. 0.750 or 0.0075

Circle the *smaller* decimal in the following pairs of decimals:

13. 0.45 or 0.7

14. 0.33 or 0.325

15. 0.25 or 0.025

16. 0.003 or 0.03

17. 0.85 or 0.090

18. 0.04 or 0.257

19. 0.05 or 0.50

20. 0.45 or 0.455

21. 0.125 or 0.025

22. 0.1 or 0.001

23. 0.600 or 0.064

24. 0.7 or 0.75

25. 0.2 or 0.04

12 PERCENTAGE

Percentage means hundredths. A percent (%) is the same as a fraction in which the denominator is 100; the numerator indicates the part of 100 being considered.

> EXAMPLE: $3\% = \dfrac{3}{100}$

In the above example, 3 parts of 100 are being considered.

When multiplying or dividing by a percent, the percent is usually changed to a decimal. *To change a percent to a decimal, remove the percent sign and divide the number by 100; that is, move the decimal point two places to the left.*

> EXAMPLE: $3\% = 100\overline{)3.00}$ or 0.03_x
> 0.03

To change a decimal to percent, multiply the decimal by 100; that is, move the decimal point two places to the right and append the percent sign.

> EXAMPLE: $0.03 \times 100 = 0_x03.\%$ or 3%

Exercise

Change the following percentages to decimals and fractions as indicated by the column headings. Reduce fractions to lowest terms.

	Decimal	Fraction
1. 8%	_____	_____
2. 15%	_____	_____
3. 90%	_____	_____
4. 20%	_____	_____

	Decimal	Fraction
5. 0.05%	_____	_____
6. 67%	_____	_____
7. 10%	_____	_____
8. 98%	_____	_____
9. 40%	_____	_____
10. 0.005%	_____	_____
11. 0.06%	_____	_____
12. 12%	_____	_____
13. 8.8%	_____	_____
14. 9.2%	_____	_____

Change the following decimals to percents:

1. 0.45 _____

2. 0.043 _____

3. 0.25 _____

4. 0.065 _____

5. 1.256 _____

6. 0.125 _____

7. 2.2 _____

8. 2.48 _____

9. 0.75 _____

10. 0.075 _____

11. 0.015 _____

12. 0.16 _____

13. 15.75 _____

14. 0.1 _____

15. 0.8 _____

16. 0.68 _____

17. 0.12 _____

18. 0.57 _____

19. 0.455 _____

20. 0.008 _____

21. 0.15 _____

22. 0.5 _____

23. 0.009 _____

24. 18.3 _____

25. 9.12 _____

13 FRACTIONS, DECIMALS, AND PERCENTAGES

Sometimes it is necessary to solve problems that contain a combination of fractions, decimals, or percentages. Such problems are solved by first converting all numbers in the problem to fractions or to decimal numbers, and then applying the rules for solving the problem. (These rules are found in Chapters 2 through 11.)

EXAMPLE: $0.4 \times \dfrac{3}{5}$

$$0.4 \times 0.6 = 0.24$$

or

$$\dfrac{\overset{2}{\cancel{4}}}{\underset{5}{\cancel{10}}} \times \dfrac{3}{5} = \dfrac{6}{25}$$

Exercise

Solve the following problems by converting the decimals or percents to fractions:

1. $10\% \times \dfrac{4}{5}$

2. $0.75 \times \dfrac{8}{9}$

3. $\dfrac{2}{3} \times 0.3$

4. $4.88 - 1\dfrac{1}{2}$

5. $7.55 \div 45\%$

6. $8\dfrac{4}{5} \div 0.2$

7. $4\dfrac{1}{4} \div 8.5$

8. $9.2 \div 5\dfrac{7}{10}$

9. $6.6 - 2\frac{7}{10}$

11. $5\frac{1}{4} \div 2\frac{1}{5}$

10. $3.8 - 2\frac{4}{5}$

12. $8.6 \div 2\frac{1}{5}$

Solve the following problems by converting the fractions or percents to decimals:

13. $0.44 + \frac{1}{50}$

20. $5\frac{1}{8} - 0.25$

14. $0.92 + 3\frac{2}{5}$

21. $5.6 \div 2\frac{4}{5}$

15. $5\frac{7}{8} + .3578$

22. $5\% \times 165$

23. $2.2 \times 68\frac{1}{2}$

16. $62\frac{3}{8} - 1.1$

24. $8 \times 2\frac{1}{2}$

17. $9\frac{2}{5} - 5.7$

25. 2% of 80

18. $0.81 \div \frac{3}{4}$

19. $4.4 \div 2\frac{1}{5}$

14 RATIO

A ratio consists of two figures separated by a colon.

EXAMPLES: 1:50   3:100

A ratio indicates that there is some relationship between the two figures. In the example cited above, the first ratio indicates that 1 is related to 50; in the second, that 3 is related to 100.

The ratio of two numbers is the quotient obtained by dividing the first by the second. Thus, *a ratio is an indicated fraction,* and the terms of the ratio are the numerator and denominator.

The value of a ratio is not changed if both terms are multiplied or divided by the same number. Multiplication and division are the only operations that can be performed on a ratio without changing its value.

When denominate numbers (3 inches, 4 gallons, 10 years) are to be written in ratio, they must be expressed in units of the same kind. For example, the ratio of 3 inches to 2 feet must be 3:24 (changing the 2 feet to 24 inches).

A fraction may be written as a ratio, and vice versa.

EXAMPLES: $\dfrac{1}{50}$ = 1:50   3:100 = $\dfrac{3}{100}$

Ratios are also expressed in their lowest terms in the same manner as are fractions, that is, by dividing both parts of the ratio by the same number.

EXAMPLE: 2:20 = 1:10

To express a percentage as a ratio, first convert it to a fraction with 100 as the denominator; for example, 25% = $^{25}/_{100}$ = 25:100. Expressed in its lowest terms, the ratio 25:100 becomes 1:4.

To change a decimal to a ratio, multiply the decimal by 100, or move the decimal point two places to the right, and use 100 as the other part (the denominator) of the ratio.

EXAMPLES: $0.87\frac{1}{2} = 87\frac{1}{2}:100$ $0.09 = 9:100$

$0.009 = 0.9:100$ $0.375 = 37.5:100$
or   or
$9:1000$ $375:1000$

When the denominator of a fraction is 10 or a multiple of 10 it may be written as a fraction, as a decimal, or as a ratio. For example, when the denominator is 10, it may be written as $\frac{1}{10}$, $\frac{3}{10}$, $\frac{5}{10}$; 0.1, 0.3, 0.5; or 1:10, 3:10, 5:10. When the denominator is 100, it may be written $\frac{1}{100}$, $\frac{2}{100}$, $\frac{8}{100}$; 0.01, 0.02, 0.08; or 1:100, 2:100, 8:100. When the denominator is 1000, it may be written as $\frac{3}{1000}$, $\frac{7}{1000}$, $\frac{9}{1000}$; 0.003, 0.007, 0.009; or 3:1000, 7:1000, 9:1000.

Exercises

Rewrite the following fractions as ratios:

1. $\frac{1}{2}$ 8. $\frac{3}{8}$

2. $\frac{2}{3}$ 9. $\frac{4}{8}$

3. $\frac{4}{5}$ 10. $\frac{5}{6}$

4. $\frac{3}{7}$ 11. $\frac{2}{5}$

5. $\frac{8}{9}$ 12. $\frac{1}{3}$

6. $\frac{45}{87}$ 13. $\frac{5}{6}$

7. $\frac{5}{9}$

Rewrite the following decimals as ratios expressed in lowest terms:

14. 0.36   18. 0.42

15. 0.5   19. 0.65

16. 0.8   20. 0.82

17. 0.01   21. 0.4

22. 0.03   24. 0.45

23. 0.25   25. 0.001

Rewrite the following percentages as ratios:

26. 1%   33. 5%

27. 10%   34. 17%

28. 0.7%
                                     35. $33\frac{1}{3}\%$
29. 0.02%

30. 0.5%   36. 2%

31. 0.8%   37. $\frac{9}{10}\%$

32. 0.06%

                                     38. $\frac{2}{5}\%$

15 PROPORTION

Proportion is a statement showing that two ratios have equivalent value. A proportion may be written as follows:

EXAMPLE: 1:50 = 2:100 or 1:50::2:100

The inner terms of the proportion are called *means,* and the outer terms are called *extremes. In any true proportion, the product of the means equals the product of the extremes:*

$$\text{Means}$$

EXAMPLES: 1:50 = 2:100

$$\text{Extremes}$$

$$1 \times 100 = 50 \times 2 \text{ or } 100 = 100$$

Extremes   Means

If the value of one term of the proportion is not known, it is commonly represented by an *x*. The value of the unknown *(x)* is found by multiplying the means and extremes.

EXAMPLE: 7:*x* = 4:28

$$4x = 7 \times 28, \text{ or } 196$$
$$x = 196 \div 4, \text{ or } 49$$

7:49 = 4:28

$$7 \times 28 = 4 \times 49$$
$$196 = 196$$

As shown above, the computation can be checked or proved by substituting for x the answer obtained and then multiplying to be certain that the product of the means equals the product of the extremes.

When the proportion is written to show the relationship of two fractions, cross-multiply either to solve for the value of an unknown or to prove the computation is correct.

EXAMPLE:
$$\frac{2}{x} = \frac{7}{49}$$
$$7x = 2 \times 49$$
$$7x = 98$$
$$x = 98 \div 7$$
$$x = 14$$

$$\frac{2}{14} = \frac{7}{49}$$
$$7 \times 14 = 2 \times 49$$
$$98 = 98$$

Exercise

Solve for x in the following proportions:

1. $6:48 = 1:x$

2. $1:50 = 20:x$

3. $7:1 = x:4$

4. $5:x = 25:500$

5. $\frac{1}{4}:\frac{1}{6} = 1:x$

6. $5:2 = x:500$

7. $5.5:100 = x:3000$

8. $0.005:0.016 = 1:x$

9. $15:40 = x:16$

10. $20,000:x = 500:1$

11. $14:28 = 1:x$

12. $20:x = 40:80$

13. $x:0.42 = 1:0.01$

14. $0.6:x = 0.25:2$

15. $x:400 = 1:500$

16. $14:80 = 6:x$

17. $x:9 = 5:20$

18. $0.4:1 = 0.2:x$

19. $0.4:1.0 = x:2.0$

20. $\frac{1}{6}:1 = \frac{1}{4}:x$

21. $x:80 = 3:12$

22. $0.3:14 = 0.6:x$

23. $0.75:x = 4:80$

24. $\frac{1}{250}:15 = \frac{1}{500}:x$

25. $\frac{1}{2}:10 = x:20$

II SYSTEMS OF WEIGHTS AND MEASURES

In Part I the basic arithmetic necessary for intelligently preparing medications for patients was reviewed. In Part II facts acquired in Part I are applied to problems encountered when the physician's order is written in one unit or system of weights and measures and the drug available is labeled in another unit or system of weights and measures.

Computation of dosage from one unit or system of weights and measures to another requires knowledge of three systems of weights and measures—metric, apothecaries', and household. The apothecaries' system is the oldest system, dating from 1617. The metric system was introduced into Europe around 1790, is considered simpler than the apothecaries' system, and is widely used throughout the world. The United States continues to use other systems, but transition to the use of the metric system is evident in the dual labeling of gauges, road signs, commercial products, and drugs. The Metric Conversion Act of 1975 commits the United States to convert to the metric system but does not specify a date by which this conversion will be completed. The metric system is the only system approved and used by the *United States Pharmacopeia (U.S.P.)*. The household system is used primarily for measuring dosages in the home; it is the least accurate of the three systems.

16 METRIC SYSTEM: WEIGHT AND VOLUME

The metric system is more accurate and flexible than other systems of weights and measures. Calculations within the metric system can be done rapidly and easily.

The metric system is based on the decimal system in which division and multiples of a unit are in ratios of tens. The units used in the metric system are as follows:

> liter (L)—volume of fluids
> gram (g)—weight of solids
> meter (m)—measure of length

Subdivisions of the units of the metric system are designated with prefixes as follows:

> deci = 0.1 of the unit
> centi = 0.01 of the unit
> milli = 0.001 of the unit

Multiples of metric units are designated with prefixes as follows:

> deka = 10 times the unit
> hecto = 100 times the unit
> kilo = 1000 times the unit

The following lists illustrate the use of prefixes that show division or multiplication of each metric unit. Although the unit of length—the meter—is not used in computation of dosage, it is used for measurements, some of which are related to the response to drug therapy and the size of areas to which drugs have been applied. This is discussed in Chapters 20 and 21. The same pattern is used for the meter as is shown for the liter and gram.

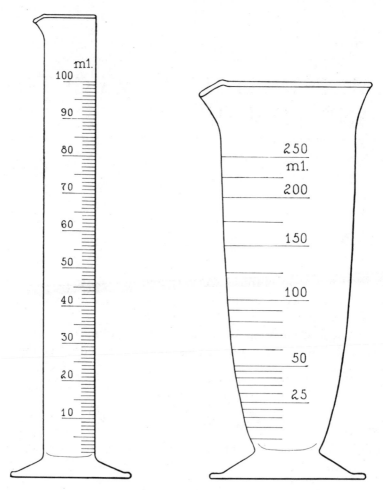

Metric measures suited to measurement of volume. Both containers are marked in milliliters. Cylindrical graduate on left is marked so that small amounts can be measured more accurately than with graduate on right. (From Hahn, A., and others: Pharmacology in nursing, ed. 15, St. Louis, 1982, The C.V. Mosby Co.)

Metric equivalents

Volume—liter (L)			Weight—gram (g)		
0.001	liter	= 1 milliliter	0.001	gram	= 1 milligram
0.01	liter	= 1 centiliter	0.01	gram	= 1 centigram
0.1	liter	= 1 deciliter	0.1	gram	= 1 decigram
10	liters	= 1 dekaliter	10	grams	= 1 dekagram
100	liters	= 1 hectoliter	100	grams	= 1 hectogram
1000	liters	= 1 kiloliter	1000	grams	= 1 kilogram

The previous lists represent complete tables of volume and weight. As a rule, nurses use only the decimals. The following tables are used frequently and should be memorized:

Units of weight

1 gram (g) = 1000 milligrams (mg)
0.001 gram (g) = 1 milligram (mg)
1 kilogram (kg) = 1000 grams (g)
0.001 kilogram (kg) = 1 gram (g)

Units of volume

1 liter (L) = 1000 milliliters (ml)
0.001 liter (L) = 1 milliliter (ml)
1 milliliter (ml) = 1 cubic centimeter (cc)

The abbreviation for gram (g) may be capitalized (Gm) in an effort to avoid confusion with the abbreviation for grain (gr). The abbreviation for meter (m) occasionally is capitalized (M).

A zero placed in front of the decimal point tends to ensure accuracy by alerting the nurse to look for a decimal point.

Exercise

Change the following units of weight in the metric system into the indicated equivalents:

1. 0.1 mg = _____ g

2. 2 g = _____ mg

3. 0.5 g = _____ mg

4. 0.3 g = _____ mg

5. 0.015 g = _____ mg

6. 2500 g = _____ kg

7. 8 mg = _____ g

8. 10 mg = _____ g

9. 5 mg = _____ g

10. 30 mg = _____ g

11. 1 mg = _____ g

12. 0.5 mg = _____ g

13. 1.2 g = _____ mg

14. 50 g = _____ mg

15. 4000 g = _____ kg

16. 0.005 g = _____ mg

17. 15 mg = _____ g

18. 2.5 g = _____ mg

19. 60 mg = _____ g

20. 0.2 mg = _____ g

21. 1 g = _____ mg

22. 0.04 mg = _____ g

23. 0.0004 g = _____ mg

24. 50 g = _____ kg

25. 0.0002 g = _____ mg

26. 50 mg = _____ g

27. 25 mg = _____ g

28. 0.008 g = _____ mg

29. 20 g = _____ mg

30. 6500 g = _____ kg

Change the following units of volume in the metric system into the indicated equivalents:

1. 14 cc = _____ ml   11. 20 ml = _____ L

2. 1 L = _____ cc   12. 0.1 L = _____ cc

3. 0.5 L = _____ ml   13. 0.4 L = _____ ml

4. 500 cc = _____ L   14. 0.75 L = _____ cc

5. 1 L = _____ ml   15. 200 cc = _____ L

6. 20 cc = _____ ml   16. 5 ml = _____ L

7. 5 ml = _____ cc   17. 0.85 L = _____ cc

8. 2 ml = _____ L   18. 30 cc = _____ L

9. 4 ml = _____ cc   19. 600 ml = _____ L

10. 250 ml = _____ L   20. 0.15 L = _____ cc

17 APOTHECARIES' SYSTEM

Although the apothecaries' system is being replaced by the metric system, it continues to be used by some physicians and in some hospitals. The following tables of equivalents should be learned by the nurse:

Volume

60 minims (ℳ) = 1 fluidram (f℥)
8 fluidrams (f℥) = 1 fluidounce (f℥)
16 fluidounces (f℥) = 1 pint (pt or O)
2 pints (pt or O) = 1 quart (qt)
4 quarts (qt) = 1 gallon (gal or C)

Weight (Troy)

60 grains (gr) = 1 dram (℥)
8 drams (℥) = 1 ounce (℥)
12 ounces (℥) = 1 pound (lb)*

When an order is written in the apothecaries' system symbols may be used. The symbol for the unit of measure is followed by the quantity, expressed in Roman numerals.† When the unit of measure is written as a word or abbreviation, the quantity is expressed in Arabic numbers and precedes the unit of measure.

EXAMPLES: ℥i = 1 dram
℥ii = 2 ounces
gr xl = 40 grains
ℳxl = 40 minims

---

*16 ounces = 1 pound avoirdupois, which is commonly used as a measure of weight in the United States.
†The exception to this is when using fractions of a unit. Then the fraction comes after the abbreviation or symbol but is in Arabic numbers; for example, ¼ grain is written gr ¼.

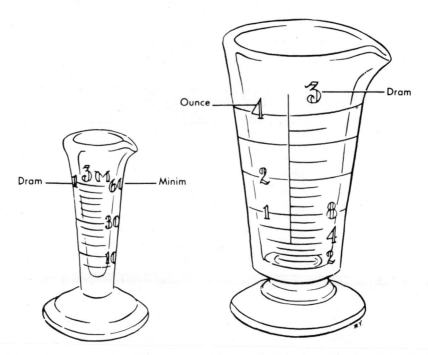

Apothecaries' measures. After dose is measured in minims, it is poured into medicine glass for administration. Minim glass is rinsed with water and this solution is also poured into medicine glass. Fluidounce measure is used to prepare larger quantities. When solution is being prepared, solute is placed in measure and water is added to make total amount of solution. (From Hahn, A., and others: Pharmacology in nursing, ed. 15, St. Louis, 1982, The C.V. Mosby Co.)

Exercise

Change the following units of volume in the apothecaries' system to the indicated equivalents:

1. ½ pint = _____ fluidounces

2. ½ fluidounce = _____ minims

3. 1 fluidram = _____ minims

4. 4 fluidrams = _____ fluidounces

5. 2 pints = _____ fluidounces

6. 2 fluidrams = _____ fluidounce

7. 1 fluidram = _____ fluidounces

8. 1 fluidounce = _____ fluidrams

9. 180 minims = _____ fluidrams

10. 1 fluidounce = _____ minims

11. 8 fluidounces = _____ pint

12. ½ fluidram = _____ minims

13. ½ fluidounce = _____ fluidrams

14. ¼ fluidounce = _____ fluidrams

15. 1 pint = _____ quart

16. 1 pint = _____ fluidounces

17. ½ pint = _____ fluidrams

18. 2 quarts = _____ gallon

19. 8 fluidrams = _____ fluidounces

Change the following units of weight in the apothecaries' system to the indicated equivalents:

1. 1 ounce = _____ drams

2. 2 drams = _____ ounce

3. 2 pounds = _____ ounces

4. 4 drams = _____ ounce

5. 1 dram = _____ grains

6. 2 ounces = _____ drams

7. 15 grains = _____ dram

8. 4 ounces = _____ drams

9. 6 drams = _____ ounce

10. ½ pound = _____ ounces

11. 6 ounces = _____ pound

12. 8 drams = _____ ounce

13. 2 drams = _____ grains

14. 30 grains = _____ dram

15. 1 ounce = _____ grains

16. ½ ounce = _____ drams

17. 120 grams = _____ drams

For each of the following units of measure, state the appropriate symbol (questions 1 through 5) or abbreviation (questions 6 through 8):

1. Ounce ⎯⎯⎯⎯   5. Minim ⎯⎯⎯⎯

2. Dram ⎯⎯⎯⎯   6. Pound ⎯⎯⎯⎯

3. Gallon ⎯⎯⎯⎯   7. Grain ⎯⎯⎯⎯

4. Pint ⎯⎯⎯⎯   8. Quart ⎯⎯⎯⎯

State the units of measure indicated by the following abbreviations or symbols:

1. ℥ ⎯⎯⎯⎯   7. qt ⎯⎯⎯⎯

2. C ⎯⎯⎯⎯   8. L ⎯⎯⎯⎯

3. O ⎯⎯⎯⎯   9. ʒ ⎯⎯⎯⎯

4. ♏ ⎯⎯⎯⎯   10. pt ⎯⎯⎯⎯

5. gr ⎯⎯⎯⎯   11. f℥ ⎯⎯⎯⎯

6. lb ⎯⎯⎯⎯   12. fʒ ⎯⎯⎯⎯

18 APPROXIMATE EQUIVALENTS: METRIC AND APOTHECARIES' SYSTEMS

Although preference for the metric system is becoming more common, the need to convert from one system to another continues to exist. Knowledge of commonly used equivalents is helpful to the nurse who must convert rapidly from one system to another. *Conversion results in an answer that is an approximate equivalent, not an equal answer.* Variations between exact and equivalent dosages may differ as much as 10%. When the need to convert dosages involves less commonly used equivalents, it is suggested that a table of approximate equivalents be consulted, such as Table 1.

It is recommended that the following equivalents be learned:

Volume

Metric system		*Apothecaries' equivalents*
1 milliliter (ml)*	=	15 minims (♏xv)
4 milliliters (ml)	=	1 fluidram (f℥i)
30 milliliters (ml)	=	1 fluidounce (f℥i)
500 milliliters (ml)	=	1 pint (O i)
1000 milliliters (ml) or 1 liter (L)	=	1 quart (1 qt)

Weight

Metric system		*Apothecaries' equivalents*
0.06 gram (g) or 60 milligrams (mg)	=	1 grain (gr i)
1 gram (g) or 1000 milligrams (mg)	=	15 grains (gr xv)
4 grams (g)	=	1 dram (℥i)
30 grams (g)	=	1 ounce (℥i)
0.45 kilogram (kg)	=	1 pound (1 lb)
1 kilogram (kg)	=	2.2 pounds (lb)

---

*Milliliters (ml) and cubic centimeters (cc) are generally accepted as equivalents.

Table 1. Approximate equivalents: metric and apothecaries' systems

Volume			Weight		
			gr	**mg**	**g**
1 fluidounce (f℥) = 30	ml (cc)		30 =	2000	= 2
$\frac{1}{2}$ fluidounce (f℥) = 15	ml (cc)		15 =	1000	= 1
			12 =	750	= 0.75
			10 =	600	= 0.6
$2\frac{1}{2}$ fluidrams (f⌬) = 10	ml (cc)		$7\frac{1}{2}$ =	500	= 0.5
2 fluidrams (f⌬) = 8	ml (cc)				
$1\frac{1}{4}$ fluidrams (f⌬) = 5	ml (cc)		5 =	300	= 0.3
			4 =	250	= 0.25
1 fluidram (f⌬) = 4	ml (cc)		3 =	200	= 0.2
45 minims (ℳ) = 3	ml (cc)		2 =	120	= 0.12
30 minims (ℳ) = 2	ml (cc)		$1\frac{1}{2}$ =	100	= 0.1
15 minims (ℳ) = 1	ml (cc)				
12 minims (ℳ) = 0.75	ml (cc)		1 =	60	= 0.06
10 minims (ℳ) = 0.6	ml (cc)		$\frac{3}{4}$ =	50	= 0.05
8 minims (ℳ) = 0.5	ml (cc)				
5 minims (ℳ) = 0.3	ml (cc)		$\frac{1}{2}$ =	30	= 0.03
4 minims (ℳ) = 0.25	ml (cc)				
3 minims (ℳ) = 0.2	ml (cc)		$\frac{1}{3}$ =	20	= 0.02
$1\frac{1}{2}$ minims (ℳ) = 0.1	ml (cc)		$\frac{1}{4}$ =	15	= 0.015
1 minim (ℳ) = 0.06	ml (cc)		$\frac{1}{6}$ =	10	= 0.010
$\frac{3}{4}$ minim (ℳ) = 0.05	ml (cc)		$\frac{1}{8}$ =	8	= 0.008
$\frac{1}{2}$ minim (ℳ) = 0.03	ml (cc)		$\frac{1}{10}$ =	6	= 0.006
			$\frac{1}{16}$ =	4	= 0.004
			$\frac{1}{20}$ =	3	= 0.003
			$\frac{1}{40}$ =	1.5	= 0.0015
			$\frac{1}{60}$ =	1	= 0.0010
			$\frac{1}{100}$ =	0.6	= 0.0006
			$\frac{1}{120}$ =	0.5	= 0.0005
			$\frac{1}{150}$ =	0.4	= 0.0004
			$\frac{1}{200}$ =	0.3	= 0.0003
			$\frac{1}{500}$ =	0.12	= 0.00012
			$\frac{1}{1000}$ =	0.06	= 0.00006

To change grams (g) to milligrams (mg), multiply by 1000, since there are 1000 milligrams in 1 gram.

EXAMPLE: 0.005 g = 5 mg

To change milligrams (mg) to grams (g), divide by 1000.

EXAMPLE: 5 mg = 0.005 g

This is not conversion from one system to another; this changes a larger denomination to a smaller or a smaller denomination to a larger, much as we change $1.00 to 100 pennies or exchange 100 pennies for $1.00. It can be seen that changing a larger denomination to a smaller denomination results in more units of the smaller denomination, and vice versa. The initial value remains unchanged.

If the physician orders the dose in grams and the medication available is in grains, the grams must be converted to grains or the grains to grams, just as German marks must be converted into French francs or French francs into American dollars.

The proportion method, discussed in Chapter 15, can be used for this purpose.

EXAMPLE A: Change 0.25 pint to milliliters.
Known (or needed) fact: 1 pint = 500 milliliters.
Establish a proportion, using the known fact as one ratio and the problem as the other ratio in the proportion. The order of the parts of each ratio must be the same, such as pints to milliliters.

$$\text{pints:milliliters} = \text{pints:milliliters}$$
$$1:500 \qquad = \qquad 0.25:x$$

Means

Extremes

$$1x = 0.25 \times 500$$
$$x = 125.\cancel{00} \text{ milliliters in 0.25 pint}$$

EXAMPLE B: Change 15 milligrams to grains.
Known fact: 60 milligrams = 1 grain.
Establish a proportion.

$$\text{milligrams:grains} = \text{milligrams:grains}$$
$$60:1 = 15::x$$
$$60x = 15$$
$$x = 15 \div 60 \text{ or } \frac{15}{60}$$
$$x = 0.25 \text{ grain or } \frac{1}{4} \text{ grain}$$

Exercise

Change the following grams to milligrams:

1. 0.01 g = _____ mg
2. 3 g = _____ mg
3. 0.016 g = _____ mg
4. 0.0015 g = _____ mg
5. 0.1 g = _____ mg
6. 0.075 g = _____ mg
7. 0.5 g = _____ mg
8. 0.05 g = _____ mg

9. 0.25 g = _____ mg
10. 0.32 g = _____ mg
11. 0.04 g = _____ mg
12. 0.0048 g = _____ mg
13. 0.64 g = _____ mg
14. 2 g = _____ mg
15. 1.5 g = _____ mg

Change the following milligrams to grams:

16. 0.5 mg = _____ g
17. 8 mg = _____ g
18. 12 mg = _____ g
19. 50 mg = _____ g
20. 340 mg = _____ g
21. 32 mg = _____ g
22. 10 mg = _____ g
23. 60 mg = _____ g

24. 2200 mg = _____ g
25. 200 mg = _____ g
26. 120 mg = _____ g
27. 16 mg = _____ g
28. 27 mg = _____ g
29. 8 mg = _____ g
30. 250 mg = _____ g

Exercise

Change the following apothecaries' units to the metric system[*]:

1. f℥ii = _____ ml

2. 120 lb = _____ kg

3. f℥iv = _____ ml

4. ♏lx = _____ ml

5. O ii = _____ ml

6. f℥iss† = _____ ml

7. ♏xxx = _____ ml

8. gr xv = _____ g

9. gr ss = _____ mg

10. ℥ii = _____ mg

11. gr xv = _____ mg

12. 7.5 lb = _____ kg

13. gr v = _____ mg

14. gr x = _____ mg

15. 180 lb = _____ kg

16. 7 lb = _____ g

17. 0.5 lb = _____ g

18. 5 lb = _____ kg

19. gr xx = _____ mg

20. 75 lb = _____ kg

Change the following metric units to the apothecaries' equivalent indicated[*]:

21. 1.5 ml = ♏ _____

22. 8 ml = f℥ _____

23. 15 ml = f℥ _____

24. 0.06 g = gr _____

25. 0.03 g = gr _____

26. 1.5 g = gr _____

27. 0.1 g = gr _____

28. 2 ml = ♏ _____

29. 500 mg = gr _____

30. 6 g = gr _____

31. 2 g = gr _____

32. 16 mg = gr _____

33. 32 mg = gr _____

34. 24 mg = gr _____

35. 75 kg = _____ lb

36. 5500 g = _____ lb

37. 20 g = ℥ _____

38. 10 kg = _____ lb

39. 8 kg = _____ lb

40. 35 kg = _____ lb

---

[*]Use of various approaches with differing equivalents may, because of the approximation, give correct answers that deviate as much as 10% from the listed answer.

†ss = one half.

19 HOUSEHOLD MEASURES

Hospitals provide calibrated medicine glasses, calibrated medicine droppers, and other measuring equipment designed to promote accurate measurement of prescribed doses. When such equipment is not available in the home, it is convenient to use household utensils to measure dosage. This requires knowledge of household equivalents and the permission of the attending physician. In a few instances, the physician may indicate that the nature of the drug, the condition of the patient, or other factors require greater accuracy of measurement. In such situations, the appropriate calibrated measuring equipment, which is available at drugstores and pharmaceutical supply houses, must be obtained.

Volume

15 drops (gtt xv) = 1 ml or 1 cc
1 teaspoonful (t) = 1 fluidram (fℨi) or 5 (4) ml*
1 tablespoonful (T) = 4 fluidrams (fℨiv)
2 tablespoonfuls (T) = 1 fluidounce (fℨi)
6 fluidounces (fℨvi) = 1 teacupful
8 fluidounces (fℨviii) = 1 glassful

Household, apothecaries', and metric equivalents

Household	Apothecaries'	Metric
1 drop =	1 minim	= 0.06 ml
1 teaspoonful =	1 fluidram	= 5 (4) ml*
1 tablespoonful =	4 fluidrams	= 15 ml
2 tablespoonfuls =	1 fluidounce	= 30 ml
1 teacupful =	6 fluidounces	= 180 ml
1 glassful =	8 fluidounces	= 240 ml

To measure a liquid, the measuring container is held in one hand (usually the left) at eye level, with the thumbnail placed on the exact calibra-

---

*A scant teaspoonful is accepted as 4 ml, whereas a filled teaspoonful is regarded as 5 ml.

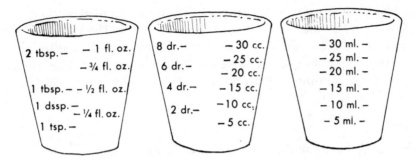

2 tbsp. —	— 1 fl. oz.
	— ¾ fl. oz.
1 tbsp. —	— ½ fl. oz.
1 dssp. —	
	— ¼ fl. oz.
1 tsp. —	

8 dr. —	— 30 cc.
6 dr. —	— 25 cc.
	— 20 cc.
4 dr. —	— 15 cc.
	— 10 cc.
2 dr. —	— 5 cc.

| — 30 ml. — |
| — 25 ml. — |
| — 20 ml. — |
| — 15 ml. — |
| — 10 ml. — |
| — 5 ml. — |

Disposable medicine glasses made of plastic material. Household, apothecaries' and metric measures are indicated. (From Hahn, A., and others: Pharmacology in nursing, ed. 15, St. Louis, 1982, The C.V. Mosby Co.)

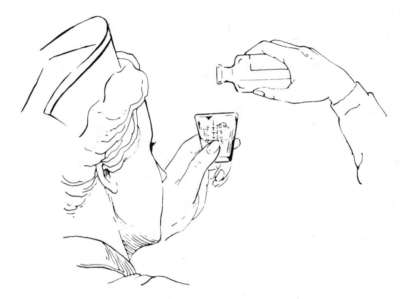

When preparing liquid dose, nurse holds measure at eye level, with thumbnail resting on calibration that marks level to which liquid will be poured.

tion that coincides with the dose to be measured. The solution tends to cling to the side of the measure, producing an elliptical curve, called the *meniscus.* The lower curve of the meniscus should rest on the calibration line of the dose being measured.

Some preparations are supplied in bottles fitted with a calibrated dropper. This contributes to accurate measurement. Considerable variation in dosage results when ordinary medicine droppers are used to measure dosage. This can be related to factors such as the size of the opening in the dropper, the angle at which the dropper is held, and the viscosity of the liquid being measured. As a rule, medications supplied with calibrated droppers should be measured only in those droppers. The label on the preparation must be read carefully because a dropper may be calibrated to release a specific number of drops per milliliter of solution. The nurse must be aware that the number of drops per milliliter may differ from the equivalents previously listed.

Exercise

Change the following units to the indicated equivalents:

1. f℥i = f℈ _____

2. f℥ii = _____ T

3. 30 ml = _____ T

4. 2 ml = ℳ _____

5. 4 ml = _____ t

6. f℈iv = _____ t

7. f℈iv = _____ T

8. f℥i = _____ T

9. 4 ml = ℳ _____

10. 15 ml = _____ T

11. 16 ml = _____ t

12. 3 cc = ℳ _____

13. $\frac{1}{4}$ t = _____ gtt

14. f℥i = _____ t

15. $\frac{1}{2}$ t = _____ gtt

16. f℥viii = _____ glassful

17. 8 ml = _____ t

18. ℳii = _____ gtt

19. 1 g = gr _____

20. ℳlx = _____ t

21. 20 cc = _____ ml

22. gtt iv = ℳ _____

23. 6 ml = _____ t

24. 180 ml = _____ cc

25. 160 cc = _____ glassful

20 METRIC SYSTEM: UNITS OF LENGTH

Metric units of length may be used to prescribe the size of an area to which medication is to be applied topically, to measure the size of wheals formed by intradermal injection of drugs, and to compare the size of skin reactions to drugs when testing for allergy to selected substances. The tuberculin test is based on this principle. Linear measurements also are used to determine the size of wounds and the size of areas saturated with drainage. Such measurements serve as a baseline to which new measurements can be compared. This information provides guidance in judging whether the size of an area has changed. Measurement of the diameter of a decubitus ulcer provides additional data about its healing and the effectiveness of the treatment being used to promote healing. Accurate measurement in units of length is superior to subjective judgment based on observation alone.

Height, length, and circumference are measured in centimeters; for example, the circumference of the head and the length of an infant are recorded in centimeters. The girth of the abdomen may be used to determine whether the amount of distention has changed and how much it has changed within a given period of time. The size of prescribed garments, such as selected abdominal binders and elastic stockings or leotards, is based on multiple measurements that are specified by the manufacturer.

Scientific instruments are calibrated in metric units of length. The sphygmomanometer is calibrated in millimeters of mercury, and the manometer of central venous pressure equipment is calibrated in centimeters of water. Pressure delivered by many mechanical breathing devices and ventilators is measured in centimeters of water. The length of tubes is also calibrated in centimeters.

The distance that a patient ambulates or travels can be recorded in metric units of length. Screening tests for vision and hearing specify the distance between the person being tested and the stimulus—a specified level of sound or a Snellen eye chart—to which he is asked to respond.

The meter is the fundamental unit of linear measure in the metric system. A meter is equivalent to 39.37 inches (39.4 inches), which is about three and a half inches longer than a yard. The prefixes used to indicate subdivisions or multiples of units of metric measures of length are the same as those listed for metric units of weight and volume on p. 57.

Length—meter (m*)

0.001	meter	= 1 millimeter (mm)
0.01	meter	= 1 centimeter (cm)
0.1	meter	= 1 decimeter (dm)
10	meters	= 1 dekameter (dam)
100	meters	= 1 hectometer (hm)
1000	meters	= 1 kilometer (km)

The above table represents a complete table of linear measure. The most frequently used metric measures of length are the kilometer, meter, centimeter, and millimeter. The centimeter and millimeter are used more frequently in the practice of nursing than are the kilometer and meter. The following list presents equivalents that are used frequently:

Units of length

1 meter (m) = 1000 millimeters (mm)
0.001 meter (m) = 1 millimeter (mm)
1 meter (m) = 100 centimeters (cm)
1 centimeter (cm) = 10 millimeters (mm)
1 millimeter (mm) = 0.1 centimeter (cm)

Exercise

Change the following units of the metric system of linear measure into the indicated equivalents:

1. 2 m = _____ mm   9. 1800 cm = _____ m

2. 10 cm = _____ mm   10. 40 mm = _____ cm

3. 100 m = _____ cm   11. 1000 mm = _____ m

4. 0.55 m = _____ cm   12. 20 cm = _____ mm

5. 28 cm = _____ mm   13. 30 mm = _____ cm

6. 450 mm = _____ m   14. 50 mm = _____ cm

7. 8 cm = _____ mm   15. 45 cm = _____ mm

8. 1725 mm = _____ cm

---

*The abbreviation for meter (m) occasionally is capitalized (M).

Solve the following problems

16. The circumference of the patient's thigh measures 57.25 centimeters; this is equivalent to _____millimeters.

17. The nurse observes drainage on a wound dressing and charts the following:

    10 PM   S: "My incision suddenly stopped hurting so much."
               O: Seropurulent drainage from wound measuring approximately 2.5 cm in diameter.
               A: Early drainage from wound.
               P: Change dressing. Reassess amount in drainage in 1 hour.

    At 11 PM, the area of drainage on the dressing is approximately 5 cm in diameter. The amount of drainage has increased by (a) _____ cm; it is (b) _____ times as large as the area of drainage recorded at 10 PM.

18. The patient complains of abdominal distention. His abdominal girth is measured at 9 AM daily. If his girth is 85 cm today and is 105 cm tomorrow, it can be said that his girth has increased by _____ cm.

19. If the patient's girth is 95 cm today and 870 mm tomorrow, would this represent a(n) _____ (increase or decrease)?

20. The nurse is to test a patient's skin reaction to a medication by applying a 0.5 cm circle of ointment containing the medication. This is the same as an area of _____ mm.

21 LINEAR UNITS OF MEASURE: METRIC-ENGLISH CONVERSIONS

The trend is to use metric units to measure length, so persons who have learned the English system will find it necessary to make conversions between the two systems. The common English linear units of measure are:

12 inches (in) = 1 foot (ft)
3 feet (ft) = 1 yard (yd)

Other units of the English system of length can be reviewed as necessary.

The following charts review common equivalents and methods of converting from one system to the other.

English system   Metric equivalents
1 inch (in) = 2.5 centimeters (cm)
1 foot (ft) = 30 centimeters (cm)
1 yard (yd) = 0.9 meters (m)
1 mile (mi) = 1.6 kilometers (km)

Metric system   English equivalents
1 kilometer (km) = 0.6 mile (mi)
1 meter (m) = 39.4 inches (in) or 1.1 yard (yd)
1 decimeter (dm) = 4 centimeters (cm)
1 centimeter (cm) = 0.4 inches (in)
1 millimeter (mm) = 0.04 inches (in)

To convert to the metric system, *multiply the English measure by its metric equivalent;* for example, to change the number of inches to centimeters, multiply by 2.5, the number of centimeters in each inch. Conversely, to change the number of centimeters to inches, divide the total number of centimeters by 2.5, the number of centimeters in an inch. Another method of converting centimeters to inches is to multiply the number of centimeters by 0.4, the number of inches in a centimeter. In other words, *to convert from the English equivalent to the metric system, multiply the known linear*

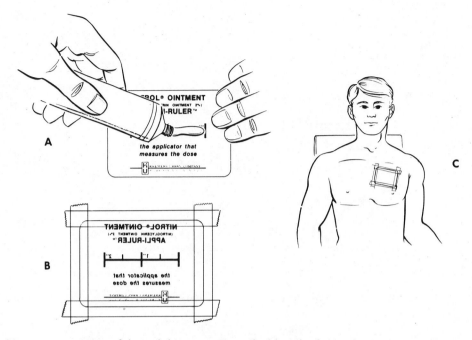

Linear measurement of desired dosage. **A,** Prescribed length of nitroglycerin ointment, 2%, is placed on APPLI-RULER™ supplied with ointment. Contact with ointment, which is absorbed through skin, should be avoided by nurse preparing dosage. **B,** Paper applicator may be used to spread ointment lightly on body and serves as dressing. Tape may be applied to ensure that applicator remains in place over ointment. **C,** Although ointment may be applied to any area of body, most patients prefer to have it applied to chest. (Courtesy, Kemers Urban Co., Milwaukee, Wis.)

measure in English by the metric unit that is equivalent. To convert to the English system from the metric system, divide the metric unit by its English equivalent. Proportions may also be used to solve problems of conversion.

Exercise

Change the following units of measure to the indicated equivalents:

1. 20 in = _____ cm

2. 3 yd = _____ m

3. 10 cm = _____ in

4. 4.5 ft = _____ cm

5. 14 mm = _____ in

6. 3 m = _____ in

7. 35 km = _____ mi

8. 80 cm = _____ ft

9. 2 in = _____ cm

10. 15 in = _____ mm

11. 2.5 mi = _____ km

12. 3 yd = _____ m

13. 50 km = _____ mi

14. 4 m = _____ yd

15. 25 cm = _____ in

16. 25 mm = _____ in

17. 17 in = _____ cm

18. 55 cm = _____ in

19. 6 in = _____ cm

20. 6 m = _____ in

21. A man who is 6 ft 2 in tall is (a) _____ cm, or (b) _____ m tall.

22. A lady who is 5 ft 5 in tall is _____ cm tall.

23. An infant who is 21 in long measures _____ cm in length.

24. If you are asked to place an inch of ointment on a particular area, this is the equivalent of _____ cm of ointment.

25. If an area of redness is measured as 1.5 in in diameter, this is equivalent to _____ cm in diameter.

26. If the abdominal girth of a person is 75 cm, it is _____ in.

27. If the abdominal girth of the person in problem 26 measures 33 in on the following day, the girth can be assessed as (a) _____ (increasing or decreasing) because 33 in is the same as (b) _____ cm.

28. The patient who is ambulated for the first time after surgery may walk a distance of 20 ft, which is the same as _____ m.

29. The following day, the patient may walk 20 m, which is the same as _____ ft.

30. If your friend says that her home is 500 mi away, this is equivalent to _____ km.

31. The highway speed limit that cars are not to exceed is usually 55 mi per hour, or _____ km per hour.

32. If the length of crutches needed is 62 in long, this is the same as _____ cm.

33. If you wish to record the following using the metric system, state the equivalents for each measure:

   a. An area of redness is 1.75 in, or _____ cm, in diameter

   b. Its location is 3 in, or _____ cm, from the shoulder

   c. Its center is elevated and white and measures ⅛ in, or _____ mm.

34. A patient in a cardiac rehabilitation program walked 2.2 miles during an exercise period. This distance is equivalent to _____ km.

35. Another person walked 6 kilometers in 2 hours. This distance is equivalent to _____ miles.

36. A piece of tubing measures ¼ inch in diameter. This is equivalent to _____ mm.

37. A length of tubing is 70 cm. This is equivalent to _____ inches.

22 CONVERSION OF TEMPERATURE FROM CELSIUS (CENTIGRADE) TO FAHRENHEIT AND VICE VERSA

Countries in which the metric system is used measure temperature in degrees Celsius. The Celsius scale was originated by Anders Celsius in 1742 in Sweden. This scale is also referred to as the centigrade scale. The Fahrenheit scale, which is used in the United States, was devised by Gabriel Fahrenheit in 1714 in Germany. The trend to convert to the metric system has increased the use of the Celsius scale in the United States, but the use of the Fahrenheit scale persists and necessitates conversion from one scale to another. The following table compares some common baselines on these two scales.

	Celsius (centigrade)	Fahrenheit
Water freezes	0°	32°
Water boils	100°	212°
Normal body temperature	37°	98.6°

Conversion from one scale to the other is done with the aid of the formulas that follow. The formula for converting degrees Celsius (centigrade) to degrees Fahrenheit is:

$$° C = \frac{5}{9} (° F - 32)$$

The formula for converting degrees Fahrenheit to degrees Celsius is as follows:

$$° F = \frac{9}{5} (° C) + 32$$

EXAMPLE A: Convert 37° C to Fahrenheit.
Use the formula:

$$°F = \frac{9}{5}(°C) + 32$$

$$°F = \frac{9}{5}(37°C) + 32$$

$$\frac{9}{5} \times 37 = \frac{333}{5} = 66.6$$

$$66.6 + 32 = 98.6$$

Therefore, 37° C is equal to 98.6° F.

EXAMPLE B: Convert 105° F to Celsius.
Substitute into the formula:

$$°C = \frac{5}{9}(°F - 32)$$

$$°C = \frac{5}{9}(105°F - 32)$$

$$\frac{5}{9} \times 73 = \frac{365}{9} \text{ or } 40.56$$

Therefore, 105° F is equivalent to 40.56° C or 40.6° C.

Exercise

Work the following problems by converting the temperatures listed as indicated.

1. 97.2° F = _____ ° C   11. 36° C = _____ ° F

2. 101.4° F = _____ ° C   12. 39.6° C = _____ ° F

3. 100.6° F = _____ ° C   13. 37.8° C = _____ ° F

4. 98.8° F = _____ ° C   14. 40° C = _____ ° F

5. 108° F = _____ ° C   15. 38.2° C = _____ ° F

6. 94° F = _____ ° C   16. 98° C = _____ ° F

7. 102° F = _____ ° C   17. 37.2° C = _____ ° F

8. 98° F = _____ ° C   18. 50° C = _____ ° F

9. 99.6° F = _____ ° C   19. 85° C = _____ ° F

10. 103.8° F = _____ ° C   20. 36.8° C = _____ ° F

III DOSAGES AND SOLUTIONS

23 INTERPRETATION AND IMPLEMENTATION OF THE PHYSICIAN'S ORDERS

Intelligent interpretation and implementation of the physician's orders is a very important nursing function. Rather than blindly following an order, the nurse must decide if the medication order is reasonable for the patient for whom it is prescribed. Correct interpretation of the physician's order is necessary if the right patient is to receive the right drug, in the right dosage, at the right time, and by the right route of administration. These are referred to as the "five rights of patients."

Legally, the nurse is permitted to administer only those medications that have been prescribed by a physician. The physician's order specifies the name of the drug, amount and frequency of the dose, and route of administration. In addition, the order shows the date the prescription was written and is signed by the prescribing physician. The form on which the physician's orders are written may vary. The following shows how one might be written (NOTE: abbreviations may also vary):

(Date)	(Time)	(Physician's orders)
1-1-84	10 AM	Give Tylenol 0.6 g q. 4 h. p.r.n. for headache.
		Dr. Spareti

Verbal orders

Policies related to the acceptance of verbal orders, including telephone orders, also differ. Institutional policies that prevent the nurse from indiscriminately accepting verbal orders protect both the patient and the nurse from potential errors, misunderstandings, and liabilities. Student nurses are rarely, if ever, permitted to accept verbal orders. Registered nurses may accept verbal orders, including those by telephone. However, many institutions have policies that discourage taking verbal orders except in emergencies. The nurse who accepts a verbal order is responsible for writing the order in the physician's order book. The order is written to indicate the date, time, name of the patient, name of the drug, dosage, method of administration, frequency of administration, name of the prescribing physician, name of the nurse accepting the order and that the order was accepted verbally. After writing the order, the nurse might sign it as follows: "Verbal order by Dr. Shakar to N. Dison." Alternatively, the nurse might write "V.O. Dr. Shakar/N. Dison." The physician is asked to sign the order at the earliest opportunity.

Transcribing the order

After the order has been received, it must be interpreted and implemented. Transcribing the order to the nursing records of the patient is usually the first step. Commonly, it is the charge nurse or the ward secretary who transcribes the orders. If the secretary transcribes the orders, the charge nurse must verify that the order is correct. After the order is transcribed, frequently referred to as "signing off the order," this is indicated on the physician's order sheet. A line may be drawn beneath the order by the person transcribing the order, and the signature of the transcriber may be placed near the end of the line. Another method may have a check mark entered at the beginning or end of the order to show that the order is now in effect. If the order is to be carried out immediately and for one time only, as occurs with "stat." orders, the nurse may indicate that the order has been carried out by placing a check mark beside the order or drawing a line beneath it and writing, "Given at 2 PM, Mary Smith."

Some hospitals use an order form that produces carbon copies. When the order has been checked off, the original copy is sent to the pharmacy to obtain a supply of the medication for the patient, and a copy remains in the physician's order book. If the order is written with triplicate copies, the original copy is sent to the pharmacy, a copy is given to the nurse responsible for administering the medication, and a copy remains in the physician's order book.

If medication cards are used, the card, completed at the time the order is transcribed, is given to the nurse responsible for administering the medication. Transfer of an order for James Brown to receive morphine sulfate, 15 mg (H), q. 4 h., to a medication card might be done as follows:

```
┌─────────────────────────────────────────────┐
│  Room 143                          12/10/83   │
│                                               │
│              BROWN, JAMES                     │
│                                               │
│        Morphine sulfate—15 mg (H)             │
│                                               │
│                 q. 4 h.                       │
│                                               │
│           9—1—5—9—1—5—9                       │
│                                               │
│                     Dr. Monroe/N. Dison       │
└─────────────────────────────────────────────┘
```

Medication or identification cards

Use of medication cards depends on the medication system employed by the particular hospital. Medication cards are not used with some medication systems. These cards are sometimes referred to as "identification cards" because they are used to identify the drug, dose, and patient. Although the size, shape, and color of the medication card used may vary, the information on the card should always state the date the order was given, name of the patient, location of the patient (room and bed numbers), name of the drug, dosage prescribed, method of administration, frequency or times of administration, and name of the prescribing physician. The name of the transcriber may be written beside the physician's name or on the back of the card. When colored medication cards are used, specific colors may be used to symbolize different times of administration. The color code used is likely to vary from one institution to another; this code is only an aid and does not change the importance of careful reading of the cards by the nurse.

Checking the transcribed order

The order may also be transcribed to the patient's nursing care plan, which may be filed in the kardex or in a notebook. Before implementing an order for the first time, it is important to check the medication card against both the care plan and the physician's order book. Thereafter, it is acceptable to check the medication card against the nursing care plan. If questions about the order arise, it should always by checked against the physician's order. The pharmacist or the physician may be consulted when appropriate.

The time at which the nurse checks the medication card against the information in the nursing care plan varies with assigned responsibilities and the particular system of communicating the plan. Some nurses do this checking when they receive report; others check all medication cards against the nursing care plans after report is received. Each nurse is responsible for making certain that the medication cards in use agree with the written orders for the medications. Assembling the medication cards in the same sequence as the medications are listed in the nursing care plan is helpful. One method of verifying that the information on the card agrees with the information in the care plan is to place the card directly beneath the order. When it is ascertained that the information is the same, the card is set aside, and the next card and order are compared.

Students who are given individual reports may check medication cards when they receive report. This permits both the student and the instructor to question information about an order that seems unclear, to seek clarification, and to communicate other essential information. The student who is not given an individual report is responsible for verifying that the information on the medication cards is correct and that a medication card is on hand for each of the prescribed medications to be administered to the patients for whom the student is responsible. Clarification must be sought whenever there is a question about interpretation of any part of a medication order. The card is checked against the original order whenever a discrepancy is found between the medication card and the nursing care plan.

Use of medication cards

The medication card is used throughout the implementation of the order. The nurse reads the medication card and compares it with the information on the drug label (1) when taking the medicine from the shelf, (2) again before the dose is removed from the container, and (3) when the container of medication is returned to its place in the medication locker. These comparisons, carried out with careful diligence, prevent errors.

Is computation necessary?

The nurse must also recognize when computation is necessary. Computation is not necessary if the dosage ordered is the same as the dosage that is available.

Avoiding interruptions while preparing the drug dosage

The undivided attention of the nurse is required during all aspects of implementing drug orders. Interruptions should be avoided if at all possible. It is considered good manners not to interrupt the nurse who is preparing medications, except in an emergency. Waiting quietly and patiently until the nurse is able to divert attention helps to prevent errors and improves working relationships. If an interruption occurs, the nurse must recheck the steps in preparing the medication.

The medication cart system

Another medication system uses a medication cart and medication kar-dexes. The medication cart contains individual drawers into which the medications for each patient are placed. The drawer is labeled with the patient's room number and name. Larger drawers in the cart are used to store equipment needed for dispensing medications to the patients, to stock supplies of frequently used medications, and to store containers too large for the smaller, individual drawers. The medication and intravenous ther-apy kardexes are kept on the countertop of the medication cart.

When the medication cart system is used, the physician's orders are transcribed into the medication kardex or the intravenous therapy kardex, whichever is appropriate. The medications may be grouped according to their route of administration. As a rule, medications that are to be given p.r.n., that is, as necessary, are listed separately from medications to be given on a timed basis. The times for administration may be indicated by a check mark placed in the appropriate column of the kardex card.

When this system is used, it is unusual to use medication cards. The order is read in the kardex (1) when taking the drug from the storage drawer, (2) after preparing the dosage to be given, and (3) before replacing the drug in the storage drawer.

A system for moving a small sliding marker, called a flag, is incorpo-rated into some kardex systems. The flag is moved to the location of the preprinted hour at which the next dosage of medication is to be given to the patient. The system of flagging depends on correct placement and use of the flag. Some nurses disregard the presence of the flag and do not posi-tion it correctly; the flag may also be positioned accidently. For these and other reasons, the flag should be regarded as a reminder that is only as reliable as its user. Many nurses recheck the entire kardex card as they administer medications to ascertain that all medications are given as pre-scribed. Other safeguards—such as checking the chart to learn when the last dosage of medication was given and to identify the drug, dose, dosage form, and patient—are observed in a system using a medication cart.

Common problems in understanding orders

Regardless of the medication system used, the nurse must understand the order perfectly before acting on it. If any aspect of the order is not understood, clarification must be sought. The physician is consulted when-ever necessary. Written orders can be confusing. For example, the symbol for dram (℥) may be written to look similar to the symbol for ounce (℥), the abbreviation for gram (g) may look like the abbreviation for grain (gr), and the numbers 4 and 7 may resemble the number 9. Other problems in the

Table 2. Abbreviations the nurse may need to interpret

Abbr.	Meaning	Abbr.	Meaning
$\bar{a}$ or a.	before	o.	every; eye
aa or $\overline{aa}$	of each	o.d.	every day; right eye
a.c.	before meals	o.h.	every hour
ad lib.	as desired; freely	o.l.	left eye
alt. h.	alternate hours	o.n.	every night
AM	in the morning; before noon	o.s.	left eye
		os	mouth
aq.	water	o.u.	both eyes
b.i.d.	twice a day	oz or ℥	ounce
b.i.n.	twice a night	$\bar{p}$ or p.	after; per
$\bar{c}$	with	p.c.	after meals
cap. or caps.	capsule	per os or p.o.	by mouth
cc	cubic centimeter	PM	afternoon; evening
comp.	compound	p.r.n.	as needed, when necessary, according to circumstances
d.	day; right		
dil.	dilute		
dist.	distilled	pulv.	powder
dr, ℨ	dram	q.	each, every
elix.	elixir	q.h.	every hour
et	and	q.i.d.	four times a day
ext.	external; extract	q. 1 h.	every one hour
fl or fld	fluid	q. 2 h.	every two hours
g	gram	q. 3 h.	every three hours
gr	grain	q. 4 h.	every four hours
gtt	drop	q. 6 h.	every six hours
H	hypodermically	q. 8 h.	every eight hours
h. or hr	hour	q. 12 h.	every twelve hours
h.s.	hour of sleep (bedtime)	q.o.d.	every other day
		q.s.	as much as needed
IM	intramuscularly	qt	quart
inj.	injection	R.	rectally
IV	intravenously	rep.	repeat
kg	kilogram	$\bar{s}$	without
L	liter	sc	subcutaneously
lb	pound	sol. or soln.	solution
liq.	liquid		
m	mix; meter	s.o.s.	if necessary
ℳ	minim	SQ	subcutaneous
mcg or μg	microgram	stat.	immediately, at once
mEq	milliequivalent	tab.	tablet
mg	milligram	tbsp or T	tablespoon
mist.	mixture; Mistogen	t.i.d.	three times a day
n.	night	tinct. or tr.	tincture
no.	number	tsp or t	teaspoon
noct.	night	U	unit
non rep.	do not repeat	ung.	ointment
O	pint		

interpretation of orders can be complex because of the illegibility of the handwriting of either the physician or the transcriber. In addition, abbreviations used in the order must be interpreted (see Table 2). If abbreviations other than the approved standard ones are used, their meaning must be verified.

Preparing the dose ordered

If a stock supply or an individual supply of medicine is used, the nurse must measure the dosage accurately. Accurate reading of the measurement of a liquid dose is facilitated by holding the measure at eye level or placing it on a shelf that is at eye level. A liquid that is to be poured is first shaken, unless otherwise specified, to suspend particles of the drug in solution. This increases the accuracy of the dosage prepared. The liquid is poured from the side of the bottle opposite the label; this helps keep the label clean and legible. After pouring the medication, the rim of the bottle may be wiped with a paper towel; this keeps the outside of the bottle clean and prevents the cap from adhering tightly to the bottle. Excess solution, if poured, must be discarded. Changes in the color, consistency, or odor of a medication require that it be returned to the pharmacy for evaluation.

If the drug is supplied in a solid dosage form, such as tablets and capsules, the cap of the bottle can be used to control the number of dosage units removed from the container. Again, if a prepared dose of medication cannot be administered, it must be discarded. The manner of disposal used must prevent any person from recovering and using the discarded drugs. Disposal of drugs that are controlled by law, such as narcotics, require the use of special procedures.

Prepackaged unit doses

The advent of prepackaged unit doses and preparation of individual doses by the pharmacist have simplified the preparation of medications by the nurse. The need to calculate dosage has been reduced. Each dose is packaged and labeled. Information on the label of a prepackaged, individual dose of medication is compared with the information contained in the prescription or in the physician's order as a method of safeguarding patient rights. In some unit dose systems, the information on the drug label serves the same purpose as does the medication card. The method of checking labeling information already described is used to compare such information. It is recommended that the individual dose remain sealed in its original container until the nurse administers it to the patient. Such packaging ensures complete identification of the drug and dosage until the drug is given. The labeling information may be imprinted on a small, wide-mouthed bottle from which the individual dose can be taken orally, on a paper enclosure that is sealed around the dose, or on a prefilled syringe. If the dose cannot be given and it remains sealed and labeled, it can be safely returned to the medication locker.

Control of drugs

Medications should never be accessible to unauthorized persons, and for this reason they are stored in a locked cupboard, room, or medication locker. Medications intended for external use should be stored separately from medications that are administered orally or parenterally. Drugs that are controlled by federal or state law must be possessed, stored, and used only in accordance with the provisions of the law. To meet the requirements of narcotics control laws, narcotic drugs are stored in a safe, locked compartment, and records are kept to document the use of these drugs. If the nurse must leave the preparation area, the medications should be placed in the locked compartment unless it is convenient to transport the medications at that time.

Administering the drug

Only the nurse who prepares a medication should administer it because the person who administers the drug is held legally responsible for giving the drug.

Before administering a medication, the nurse should determine when the patient last received that medication. This can be verified by checking the patient's chart. The medication card, as discussed before, is used to identify the dosage until it has been taken by the patient. It serves to identify the patient and is used to record administration of the medication. It can also be used to verify that the chart, the number of the room, the bed number, and the patient's name are correct and correspond to the information on the medication card. When the medication cart system is used, the kardex provides the same information as a medication card.

The nurse who does not know the patient should ask him to state his name rather than call him by name or ask, "Are you Mr. Brown?" The patient might misunderstand and respond to a name other than his own. Identification of the patient is established by checking the information on the identification bracelet worn by the patient. A second bracelet that is color-coded can be used to alert the nurse to known allergies of the patient. Although it seems logical to use a red identification bracelet to indicate allergies, other schemes for color-coding are sometimes used; this emphasizes the importance of reading the information contained on the bracelets. The bracelet may incorporate a transparent window behind which may be placed an insert on which the patient's allergies can be written. This provides a mechanism for protecting the patient from receiving potentially harmful drugs.

The nurse who implements a drug order must know the patient and the drug. Only then will the nurse be able to recognize whether the order is a reasonable one and know the precautions needed, contraindications, expected effects, and adverse reactions that may occur. For example, the nurse who must implement the drug order for James Brown (see previous boxed order) and who knows that it is unusual to give morphine sulfate every 4 hours should question whether this order was intended to be a q. 4 h. p.r.n. order. The drug order may be reasonable for the patient who has intractable pain caused by a terminal disease. The dosage of morphine sulfate, 15 mg, should be questioned if Mr. Brown is a small, frail, elderly man. The nurse should also question an order to repeat administration of an addicting drug this regularly and frequently. Knowing that morphine causes depression of the central nervous system, the nurse would observe, assess, and record the respiration as well as the level of consciousness of the patient. Knowledge that drugs depressing respiration are usually withheld if the respirations decrease to 12 or fewer per minute or if the respirations become ineffective should guide the nurse in withholding the drug. The nurse would be aware of the need to assess the heart action by listening to the apical pulse, if the order is for a derivative of digitalis. Knowing that digitalis slows and strengthens the beat of the heart influences the nurse to take an apical pulse and to withhold the drug if the heart rate has slowed to 60 or fewer beats per minute. Aware of the expected action of digitalis, the nurse would consult the physician before repeating the medication if the heart rate increased markedly or became weaker.

Charting

As soon as the nurse has administered the drug, the name of the drug, the dosage given, the route of administration, and the time when given must be charted on the patient's hospital record. Effects of the drug are assessed and recorded and, if unusual, are reported.

Times of administration

Times at which medications are administered vary from one hospital to another and even from one nursing unit to another. The schedule used is influenced by many factors. The time interval for a q. 4 h. medication might mean that the medication will be given at 8—12—4—8 in one hospital but at 9—1—5—9 in another; a schedule of 7—11—3—7 might be preferred by an outpatient. Table 3 suggests time patterns that could be used if meals are served at 7:30 AM, 11:30 AM, and 5:30 PM. A q. 4 h. order

Table 3. Suggested times for drug therapy*

Abbreviation	Interpretation	Time of administration
a.c.	before meals	7–11–5
b.i.d.	twice a day	9–7
p.c.	after meals	9–1–7
p.r.n.	whenever necessary	dose may be repeated according to stated time interval
q.d.	every day	9 AM
q.h.	every hour	7–8–9–10, and so on
q. 2 h.	every 2 hours	7–9–11, and so on
q. 3 h.	every 3 hours	6–9–12–3
q. 4 h.	every 4 hours	8–12–4–8
q. 6 h.	every 6 hours	6–12–6–12
q.i.d.	four times a day	9–1–4–7
s.o.s.	if necessary	
stat.	immediately	

From Dison, N.G.: Clinical nursing techniques, ed. 4, St. Louis, 1979, The C.V. Mosby Co.
*These are the suggested hours for drug administration if meals are served at 7:30 AM, 11:30 AM, and 5:30 PM.

for medication should not be confused with a q.i.d. order. The latter is to be given just four times in a 24-hour period; a q. 4 h. medication is given at 4-hour intervals throughout the 24-hour period. In implementation, a q. 4 h. order differs also from a q. 4 h. p.r.n. order. The latter indicates with the abbreviation p.r.n. that the drug can be given "if necessary" but not more often than every 4 hours (see Table 2).

Medications should be given at approximately the same time each day. The time at which medication is received is likely to be important to the patient, so he needs to know when deviation from the time schedule is permissible. It is suggested that a variation of no more than 15 minutes before or after the stated time for administration be allowed. Unless extenuating circumstances exist, a total time deviation of one-half hour is reasonable for most drugs that are administered by the nurse. The importance of administering the drug at the specified time varies with the nature and the purpose of the drug. The nurse who understands the patient and the action of the medication can exercise discretion about the urgency of administering a drug at a stated time. Some variation in time of administration is allowed for most drugs, even though the dosage is titrated by the blood levels of the drugs. Understanding that the drug prescribed exerts its action only when a certain blood level of the drug is maintained assists the nurse in deciding whether to awaken the patient to take the medication. A few drugs, such as those used to treat myasthenia gravis, must be administered at precise times and time intervals to maintain desired effects. The amount of time variation allowed for administering a vitamin preparation may be considerably more than that allowed for some other medications. Knowledge of the effects of drugs is necessary in determining the desirability of establishing and maintaining precise schedules for their administration.

There are times when the nurse must delay the administration of a drug, in view of the nursing assessment of the patient, until it can be determined if the physician wishes the drug to be administered or to be withheld. The decision to withhold a drug, even for a short time, must be based on understanding of the drug, the patient, and other influencing factors. The nurse who assumes the responsibility of administering medication must accept the obligation of obtaining and using knowledge about the drug and the patient intelligently.

Teaching

The nurse has multiple opportunities for teaching patients about their medications. This role may be shared with the physician and clinical pharmacist. Information helps many patients to accept drug therapy. It is common procedure to provide patients with facts such as the name, purpose, and expected effects of medications. In addition, patients should be informed of side effects that occur frequently, as well as actions that should be taken if such side effects occur. It is helpful to provide this information in written form if the medication is to be continued at home.

Discretion is used in determining the amount and kind of information that is conveyed to an individual and the manner in which it is presented. For example, any patient who is given a drug that contains a dye that discolors the urine must be told of this effect to avoid alarming the patient unnecessarily. Patients are also warned of side effects that could jeopardize their safety, such as the dizziness or light-headedness that commonly occurs after the administration of narcotics. The patient who is to continue medication therapy at home must know the signs and symptoms that indicate that he should contact the physician, the actions to take until he can obtain the advice of the physician, and whether or not to withhold the drug. Use of investigational drugs requires that the patient be fully informed; this is controlled by research protocol and laws.

The patient who is to continue drug therapy at home finds it helpful to have opportunities to learn to administer the medication under supervision during hospitalization. To do this, the patient needs considerable information, which can be provided in the form of a written plan that includes the name of the drug, its color (when appropriate), the dosage to be taken at specified times, and other helpful information. Some patients find it worthwhile to use a checklist, whereas others devise their own means of remembering the times at which to take medication. Skills in dispensing and administering the drugs are practiced until the patient develops the proficiency required for safe administration. Learning to measure and inject insulin usually requires considerable information and multiple opportunities to observe and practice the needed skills. Practice sessions allow the nurse to teach, coach, and supervise the patient and to determine the level of competence that has been achieved. The nurse may, with the patient's approval, make referrals to community agencies that will assist the patient with medication therapy at home.

Acquiring the necessary information and skill in medication therapy requires that information and practice be provided as early as possible. Planning and working with the patient and coaching him, as necessary, enables the patient to learn more efficiently and effectively and frees him from being dependent on others to manage the medication therapy. Ideally, such teaching begins very early in the delivery of health care and is individualized appropriately.

Exercise

1. The physician orders meperidine, 75 mg (IM). The prepared unit dose is labeled, "Meperidine, 75 mg in 1.5 ml." (a) How much solution should be given for the patient to receive 75 mg? (b) What does the abbreviation IM mean?
2. The physician orders neomycin, 0.5 g (p.o.). The container of tablets is labeled, "Neomycin, 0.5 g." (a) How many tablets are needed for the correct dose? (b) How is this drug to be administered?
3. The physician orders atropine, 0.4 mg (s.c.). The multidose container is labeled, "Atropine sulfate, 0.4 mg in 1 ml." (a) How many cc should the nurse withdraw? (b) How is the drug to be given?
4. The physician's order is for phenobarbital, 30 mg q.i.d. The label on the tablet reads, "Phenobarbital, 30 mg." (a) How many tablets are needed for each dose? (b) How often is this drug to be administered? (c) At what times would it be administered in the clinical agency in which you practice?
5. The physician orders Darvon, plain, 32 mg q. 6 h. The capsules are labeled, "Darvon, 32 mg." (a) How many capsules are needed to give the dose ordered? (b) How often is this dose to be repeated?
6. The physician orders Darvon Compound-65, cap. i, q.3–4 h. p.r.n. (a) How many capsules of a preparation labeled "Darvon Compound-65" are needed for one dose? (b) What is the most frequent time interval at which the dose can be repeated? (c) What does the abbreviation p.r.n. mean?

7. The physician prescribes heparin, 5000 U (IV) stat. The drug is labeled, "Heparin, 5000 U/ml." (a) What amount of heparin solution should be prepared for the dose ordered? (b) What route of administration is to be used? (c) When is the dose to be given? (d) Is the order to be repeated? (e) What does the abbreviation U mean? (f) What is the policy of your employer (or school) concerning whether the nurse may give this drug?

8. The physician prescribes Maalox, ℥ii, q. 2 h., and milk, 100 cc alt. h. (a) What is the amount of Maalox that is to be administered for each dose? (b) How often is the Maalox to be administered? (c) When is the milk to be given?

9. The physician orders aluminum phosphate, ℥i, ½ h. a.c. (a) What is the dose that should be prepared? (b) When is the drug to be given?

10. The physician orders Lugol's sol., gtt x, t.i.d. (a) Is this drug to be given in the solid or the liquid form? (b) How much drug is to be given for each dose? (c) How often is the drug to be given?

11. The physician's order reads as follows:

Aspirin
Bicarbonate of soda } gr x $\overline{aa}$ q. 3–4 h. p.r.n.

(a) How much aspirin is to be given? (b) How much bicarbonate of soda is to be given?

12. The physician orders aminophylline suppositories, gr viiss (R.) stat. and non rep. (a) What does the abbreviation R. mean? (b) What does the abbreviation non rep. indicate to the nurse? (c) How much drug should each suppository contain?

13. The physician writes an order stating, "Neosynephrine ¼%, gtt ii, o.d., b.i.d. (a) What does the abbreviation gtt stand for? (b) Which eye is to be treated? (c) How often is the treatment to be done? (d) What abbreviation might be used to indicate that both eyes are to be treated?

14. Your neighbor shows you the label on her prescription medication that reads, "Take one capsule 4 times daily for 7 days. Tetracycline 250 mg," and asks you when she ought to take the capsules. What is the major principle that she needs to understand to select the times that would allow the medicine to have its maximum effect and that would fit into her time schedule?

15. Susan Z. is to continue taking the drug lithium carbonate at 12-hour intervals when she is discharged from a psychiatric unit. These time intervals are important because the level of drug in the blood affects the quality of control of symptoms. (a) What would you tell Susan about lithium levels? (b) How might planning facilitate adherence to a

schedule of home medication that requires 12-hour intervals between doses? (c) What method(s) could be used to allow Susan to learn to take her own medication before leaving the institutional setting? (d) Whose responsibility is it to determine that Susan has been given the opportunity to learn acceptable medication practices?

16. After Susan has taken lithium for several days, she asks you what she should do if ever she is away from home and finds that she has depleted her drug supply. What are some possible alternatives for consideration in discussion of this problem?

17. Two months after Susan is discharged from the hospital, the level of lithium in her blood indicates that an increase in dosage is needed. The physician increases the dosage by two capsules each day and tells her that she may alter the times at which she takes a particular amount of drug if the increased dosage causes symptoms of nausea or diarrhea. Susan does not understand how the drug amount and schedule is to be altered. If she is now taking six capsules of lithium daily instead of the previous dose of four capsules daily, what can you suggest, knowing that maintaining the blood levels is essential?

18. The physician writes the following take-home prescriptions for a patient:

> Nefedipine, 10 mg t.i.d.
> Isordil, 10 mg q.i.d.
> Tenormin, 50 mg q.d.
> Trans-derm—nitro 5, (1) q.d.
> Colace, 100 mg cap. (1) q.d.

Make a time schedule for the patient to follow in taking these medications. Assume that the patient will be returning to a job that extends from 8 AM to 4 PM. Plan the schedule so that the medications are evenly distributed without the patient having to take medicine more than three times a day.

19. The physician orders Darvon N-100, tabs.i, to be given q. 3–4 h. p.r.n. for severe muscle pain. (a) How many tablets of the drug are to be administered? (b) What is the name of the prescribed drug? (c) How often may the dose be repeated?

20. You are using prepackaged unit doses of Tylenol. Each tablet comes individually wrapped and is labeled, "Tylenol, 0.6 g tablets." If you have prepared this medication, under what circumstances can it be replaced in the patient's individual supply of medication?

24 COMPUTATION OF DOSAGE

When the dose prescribed is in milligrams and the dose available is in grams or vice versa

If the dosage ordered by the physician is in milligrams and the dosage unit available is in grams, or vice versa, it is necessary to change one of the units so that both units are stated in the same (equal) unit of measurement. It is more logical to change to the unit of measurement stated on the label because this indicates the amount of drug contained in one dosage unit, that is, in one tablet, capsule, or milliliter. The label, "Morphine sulfate, 16 mg," indicates that each tablet in the container is equal to 16 mg of morphine sulfate. There are 1000 mg in each gram as discussed in Chapter 16. Grams are converted to milligrams by multiplying the number of grams by 1000, which is the same as moving the decimal point three places to the right. Any one of several methods may be used to solve the problem of how much drug is needed to administer the prescribed dose.

EXAMPLE: The physician prescribes 0.008 g of morphine sulfate. Tablets available (on hand) are labeled 16 mg morphine sulfate per tablet.

Regardless of the method used to solve this problem, the prescribed dose (0.008 g) must be changed to the unit of measurement stated on the label (mg). Changing grams to milligrams is done by multiplying grams by 1000:

$$0.008 \text{ (g)} \times 1000 \text{ (mg)} = 8 \text{ mg}$$

METHOD 1. One method of establishing a proportion is to use the information on the label of the drug as one part of the proportion and the dosage prescribed as the other part of the proportion. Using the example problem, the label of the drug states that there are 16 mg in each tablet, and the physician's prescribed dose is 0.008 g or 8 mg. The proportion may be established as follows:

Label side of the proportion   Dose prescribed

$$16 \text{ (mg)}:1 \text{ (tab.)} = 8 \text{ (mg)}:x \text{ (tab.)}$$

Means

Extremes

$$16x = 8$$
$$x = 8 \div 16$$
$$x = 0.5 \text{ or } \tfrac{1}{2} \text{ tab. of morphine sulfate, 16 mg per tablet}$$

When this method of establishing a proportion is used, the parts of each ratio must be placed in the same order, with the known facts from the label listed on one side of the proportion and the desired or prescribed dose on the other side of the proportion.

METHOD 2. After 0.008 g is changed to 8 mg, a proportion can be established, using known facts. The proportion must be stated so that the parts of each ratio are in the same order. It is usual to state a proportion in terms of small:large = small:large. To establish the proportion in this sequence, it is necessary to determine whether the dose prescribed is smaller or larger than the dose that is available. It is known that there are 16 mg in one tablet of the prescribed drug. The dose prescribed is 8 mg, less than the 16 mg available in a single tablet. The proportion can be established as follows:

$$\text{small}:\text{large} = \text{small}:\text{large}$$
$$\text{milligrams}:\text{milligrams} = x \text{ (tab.)}:1 \text{ (tab.)}$$
$$8 \text{ (mg)}:16 \text{ (mg)} = x \text{ (tab.)}:1 \text{ (tab.)}$$

Means

Extremes

$$16x = 8$$
$$x = 8 \div 16$$
$$x = 0.5 \text{ or } \tfrac{1}{2} \text{ tab. of morphine sulfate, 16 mg per tab-}$$

let, is needed to give 8 mg of morphine sulfate

METHOD 3. A third method of solving this problem is to substitute the known information into the following formula:

100

$$\frac{\text{dosage desired (to give the prescribed dose)}}{\text{dosage available (in each tablet or dosage unit)}} \times 1 \text{ (tab.)} =$$

number of tablets needed to give the dose prescribed

Solve the problem; then label the answer completely:

$$\frac{8 \text{ (mg prescribed)}}{16 \text{ (mg in 1 tab.)}} \times 1 \text{ (tab.)} =$$

0.5 or $\frac{1}{2}$ tab. of morphine sulfate, 16 mg. per tablet

Regardless of the method used to solve the problem, it is always wise to determine if the answer seems reasonable: 8 mg is smaller than 16 mg, and it seems reasonable to expect that 0.5 or $\frac{1}{2}$ of 16 will be equal to 8.

Exercise

Solve the following problems for correct number of tablets or capsules to be administered:

1. The physician orders acetylsalicylic acid, 600 mg. The dose on hand is 0.3 g per tablet.
2. The physician orders sodium salicylate, 0.6 g. The dose on hand is 300 mg per tablet.
3. The physician orders morphine sulfate, 5 mg. The dose on hand is in 0.015 g tablets.
4. The physician orders ascorbic acid, 0.05 g. The dose on hand is 25 mg per tablet.
5. The physician orders tetracycline, 0.75 g. The dose on hand is 250 mg capsules.
6. The physician orders calcium gluconate, 1 g. The dose on hand is 500 mg per tablet.
7. The physician orders Diuril, 0.5 g. The dose on hand is 250 mg per tablet.
8. The physician orders Benadryl, 50 mg. The dose on hand is 0.025 g per capsule.
9. The physician orders digitoxin, 0.0002 g. The dose on hand is 0.1 mg per tablet.
10. The physician orders meprobamate, 0.2 g. The dose on hand is 400 mg per tablet.
11. The physician orders codeine sulfate, 15 mg. The dose on hand is 0.03 g per tablet.

12. The physician orders atropine sulfate, 0.0006 g. The dose on hand is 0.4 mg per tablet.
13. The physician orders ephedrine, 100 mg. The dose on hand is 0.05 g per tablet.
14. The physician orders novobiocin, 0.75 g. The dose on hand is 250 mg capsules.
15. The physician orders ascorbic acid, 0.2 g. The dose on hand is 100 mg tablets.
16. The physician orders kanamycin, 1 g. The dose on hand is in 500 mg capsules.
17. The physician orders tetracycline, 0.25 g. The dose on hand is in 250 mg capsules.
18. The physician orders penicillin, 1 g. The dose on hand is in 125 mg tablets.
19. The physician orders novobiocin, 0.5 g. The dose on hand is in 250 mg capsules.
20. The physician orders Gantrisin, 2 g. The dose on hand is in 500 mg tablets.
21. Carbamazepine (Tegretol), 0.6 g, is ordered. The medication is available in 200 mg tablets.
22. The total daily dose of calcium carbonate is to equal 7.8 g/day. If this drug is available in 650 mg tablets, how many tablets will be needed each day?
23. Acetohexamide (Dymelor) is to be given in two divided doses daily. If the total daily dose is 1.5 g and the available tablets contain 250 mg of the drug, how many tablets should be used for each dose?
24. An initial dose of tolbutamide (Orinase), 2 g, is ordered. The tablets on hand are labeled, "Each tablet contains 250 mg tolbutamide." How many tablets are needed for the initial dose?
25. Dihydroxyaluminum aminoacetate (Robalate), 0.5 g, is ordered after meals and at bedtime. Assuming three meals, this amount is equal to how many 500 mg chewable tablets *daily?*

25 COMPUTATION OF DOSAGE

When the dosage ordered by the physician is larger or smaller than the dose per tablet

USING THE METRIC SYSTEM

If the physician orders 0.015 g of phenobarbital and the dose on hand is labeled, "one tablet contains 0.06 g," the problem can be solved in one of the following ways.

METHOD 1. State the proportion, using the information on the label as one part of the proportion and the desired dose as the other part of the proportion.

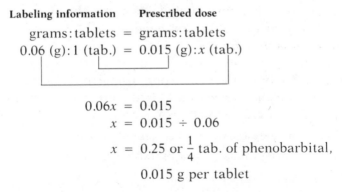

Labeling information   Prescribed dose

grams:tablets = grams:tablets

0.06 (g):1 (tab.) = 0.015 (g):x (tab.)

$$0.06x = 0.015$$
$$x = 0.015 \div 0.06$$
$$x = 0.25 \text{ or } \frac{1}{4} \text{ tab. of phenobarbital,}$$

0.015 g per tablet

To divide the tablet, the nurse may dissolve it in ℥iv of water and give ℥i, a fourth of the amount in which the tablet was dissolved. Preparation of a liquid form requires considerable knowledge of the drug preparation, for the drug may be insoluble in water or may be unstable in solution; also, the destruction of special coatings may destroy the effectiveness of the drug. *When the prescribed dose is less than the available dosage form, it is usually advisable to consult the pharmacist who will, when possible, prepare a liquid form.*

METHOD 2. State the proportion in terms of small is to large as small is to large.

$$small:large = small:large$$
$$grams:grams = tablets:tablets$$
$$0.015 \, (g):0.06 \, (g) = x \, (tab.):1 \, (tab.)$$

$$0.06x = 0.015$$
$$x = \frac{0.015}{0.06} = \frac{0.015}{0.060} = \frac{1}{4} \text{ tab. of phenobarbital, gr } \frac{1}{2} \text{ per tablet}$$

METHOD 3. Substitute into the following formula:

$$\frac{\text{desired dose}}{\text{available dose}} \times 1 \, (tab.) =$$

number of tablets needed to administer prescribed dose

$$\frac{0.015 \, (g)}{0.06 \, (g)} \times 1 \, (tab.) = \frac{0.015}{0.060} \times 1 = \frac{1}{4} \text{ tab. of phenobarbital, 0.06 g per tablet}$$

USING THE APOTHECARIES' SYSTEM

The physician orders codeine sulfate, gr ⅛, and the nurse has on hand gr ½ tablets. It is immediately known that the amount to be given (gr ⅛) is smaller than the tablets on hand (gr ½). The problem and proportion would be set up as follows:

METHOD 1. Establish the proportion, using the information on the label as one ratio and the desired dose as the other ratio of the proportion. (See Chapter 6 for dividing fractions.)

Label side of the proportion   **Desired (prescribed) dose**

$$grains:tablets = grains:tablets$$
$$\frac{1}{2} \, (gr):1 \, (tab.) = \frac{1}{8} \, (gr):x \, (tab.)$$

$$\frac{1}{2}x = \frac{1}{8}$$
$$x = \frac{1}{8} \div \frac{1}{2} = \frac{1}{8} \times \frac{2}{1}$$
$$x = \frac{2}{8} \text{ or } \frac{1}{4} \text{ tab. of codeine sulfate, gr } \frac{1}{2} \text{ per tablet}$$

METHOD 2. Establish the proportion, using small is to large as small is to large.

small:large = small:large
grain:grain = tablet:tablet

$\frac{1}{8}$ (gr):$\frac{1}{2}$ (gr) = x (tab.):1 (tab.)

$$\frac{1}{2}x = \frac{1}{8} \times 1 \text{ or } \frac{1}{8}$$

$$x = \frac{1}{8} \div \frac{1}{2} \text{ or } \frac{1}{8} \times \frac{2}{1}$$

$$x = \frac{2}{8} \text{ or } \frac{1}{4} \text{ tab. of codeine sulfate, gr } \frac{1}{2} \text{ per tablet}$$

METHOD 3. Substitute into the following formula:

$$\frac{\text{dosage desired}}{\text{dosage available}} \times 1 \text{ (tab.) =}$$

number of tablets needed to administer the prescribed dosage

$$\frac{^{1}/_{8}}{^{1}/_{2}} \times 1 = \frac{1}{8} \div \frac{1}{2} \times 1 = \frac{1}{8} \times \frac{2}{1} \times 1 =$$

$$\frac{2}{8} \text{ or } \frac{1}{4} \text{ tab. codeine sulfate, gr } \frac{1}{2} \text{ per tablet}$$

Exercise

Solve each of the following problems to find how many tablets or capsules are needed to provide the dosage prescribed:

1. The physician orders Colace, 100 mg q.d. Each capsule contains 50 mg.
2. The physician orders 60 mg of codeine. The dose on hand is 30 mg tablets.
3. The physician orders atropine sulfate, gr $^{1}/_{150}$. The dose on hand is gr $^{1}/_{100}$ tablets.
4. The physician orders 1.5 mg of Dilaudid (hydromorphinone hydrochloride). The dose on hand is 3 mg tablets.
5. The physician orders scopolamine, gr $^{1}/_{300}$. The dose on hand is gr $^{1}/_{200}$ tablets.
6. The physician orders 2 mg of dihydromorphinone. The dose on hand is 3 mg tablets.
7. The physician orders 60 mg of codeine. The dose on hand is 15 mg tablets.

8. The physician orders apomorphine, gr $\frac{1}{30}$. The dose on hand is gr $\frac{1}{10}$ tablets.

9. The physician orders potassium iodide, 600 mg q. 6 h. The enteric-coated tablets on hand each contain 300 mg. How many tablets are administered in each dose?

10. An initial dose of 500 mg of aminophylline is ordered. The tablets on hand are 100 mg.

11. The physician orders atropine, 300 μg.* The dose on hand is 1.2 mg tablets.

12. The physician orders morphine sulfate, gr $\frac{1}{4}$. The dose on hand is gr $\frac{1}{6}$ tablets.

13. The physician orders 5 mg of morphine. The dose on hand is 15 mg tablets.

14. The physician orders sodium bicarbonate, 0.64 g. The dose on hand is 0.32 g tablets.

15. The physician orders atropine, gr $\frac{1}{200}$. Tablets on hand are labeled gr $\frac{1}{150}$.

16. The physician orders acetylsalicylic acid, gr xx. The dose on hand is gr v tablets.

17. The physician orders Gantrisin (sulfisoxazole) 6 g/day in four divided doses. How many tablets are needed for each dose if each tablet contains 500 mg?

18. The physician orders atropine sulfate, 0.2 mg. Available tablets are labeled 0.4 mg.

19. The physician orders chloral hydrate, gr xv. The dose on hand is in capsules, gr $3\frac{3}{4}$.

20. The physician orders digitalis, gr ss. The dose on hand is gr iss tablets.

21. The physician orders aspirin, gr x. The dose on hand is tablets, gr v.

22. The physician orders morphine, gr $\frac{1}{4}$ (H). Available tablets are labeled gr $\frac{1}{6}$.

23. The physician orders atropine sulfate, gr $\frac{1}{120}$. Available tablets are labeled gr $\frac{1}{100}$.

24. The physician orders 1000 mg nafcillin q. 6 h. If each capsule contains 250 mg of the drug, how many capsules are given for each dose?

25. The physician orders phenobarbital, gr iss. The dose on hand is gr $\frac{1}{2}$ tablets.

26. The physician orders 0.6 mg of scopolamine. Tablets on hand are labeled 1.2 mg.

27. The physician orders 10 mg of morphine. Tablets on hand are labeled 15 mg.

---

*1 μg (microgram) = $\frac{1}{1000}$ mg.

28. The physician orders 400 μg* of atropine. Tablets on hand are labeled 600 μg.
29. The physician orders thiamine chloride, 100 mg. The dose on hand is 25 mg tablets.
30. Aquamephyton (phytonadione), 15 mg, is ordered to be given stat. Each tablet contains 5 mg.

---

*1 μg (microgram) = $\frac{1}{1000}$ mg.

26 COMPUTATION OF DOSAGE

When the physician orders a dose in one system and the dose on hand is in another system

When the physician orders a dose in one system and the dose on hand is supplied in another system (such as metric and apothecaries' or vice versa), *it is necessary to convert the dose ordered into the same system as the dose that is supplied or vice versa.* It is wise to convert the dose ordered into that on hand. Although the fact that gr i is actually equivalent to 0.0648 g should not be overlooked, when converting, it is permissible to use the equivalent 0.06 (some use 0.064 or 0.065) in place of the more exact figure. *As a rule, 10% greater or less than the exact figure is permissible.* When the dose must be measured exactly, the pharmacist computes the dosage.

If, for example, the physician orders atropine sulfate, gr $\frac{1}{150}$, and the dose on hand is 0.0006 g, it is necessary to convert the grains to grams or vice versa before computing the problem. Both the dose ordered and the dose on hand must be in the same system before the problem can be worked. (See Chapter 18.)

After recalling that 0.06 g is equivalent to gr i, the proportion is set down as follows:

grams:grains = grams:grains

$$0.06 \text{ (g)}:1 \text{ (gr)} = x \text{ (g)}:\frac{1}{150} \text{ (gr)}$$

$$x = 0.06 \times \frac{1}{150}$$

$$x = \frac{0.06}{150} = 150\overline{)0.0600}^{0.0004}$$
$$\underline{600}$$

$x = 0.0004$ g, which is equivalent to gr $\frac{1}{150}$

With the knowledge that gr $\frac{1}{150}$ is equivalent to 0.0004 g or that each dose of atropine will be either gr $\frac{1}{150}$ or 0.0004 g, the problem can be solved as follows:

METHOD 1. The proportion may be stated, using the labeling information as one part of the proportion.

   Labeling information   **Desired dose**

$$\text{gram:tablet} = \text{gram:tablet}$$
$$0.0006 \text{ (g)}:1 \text{ (tab.)} = 0.0004 \text{ (g)}:x \text{ (tab.)}$$
$$0.0006x = 0.0004$$
$$x = \frac{0.0004}{0.0006} = \frac{2}{3} \text{ tab. of atropine sulfate, } 0.0006 \text{ g per tablet}$$

METHOD 2. A proportion stating that small is to large as small is to large may be used.

$$\text{small:large} = \text{small:large}$$
$$\text{grams:grams} = \text{tablets:tablets}$$
$$0.0004 \text{ (g)}:0.0006 \text{ (g)} = x \text{ (tab.)}:1 \text{ (tab.)}$$
$$0.0006x = 0.0004 \div 0.0006$$
$$x = \frac{4}{6} \text{ or } \frac{2}{3} \text{ tab. of atropine sulfate, } 0.0006 \text{ g per tablet}$$

METHOD 3. Substitute into the following formula:

$$\frac{\text{desired dose}}{\text{available dose}} \times 1 \text{ (tab.)} =$$

            number of tablets needed to administer the dose prescribed

$$\frac{0.0004}{0.0006} \times 1 \text{ (tab.)} = \frac{4}{6} \text{ or } \frac{2}{3} \text{ tab. of atropine sulfate, } 0.0006 \text{ g per tablet}$$

If working with grains instead of grams is preferred, the conversion proportion would be the following:

$$\text{grams:grains} = \text{grams:grains}$$
$$0.06 \text{ (g)}:1 \text{ (gr)} = 0.0006 \text{ (g)}:x \text{ (gr)}$$
$$0.06x = 0.0006$$
$$x = \frac{0.0006}{0.06} = \frac{\overset{1}{\cancel{0.0006}}}{\underset{100}{\cancel{0.0600}}} = \frac{1}{100} = \text{gr } \frac{1}{100}$$

or

$$\frac{0.0006}{0.6} \times \frac{1000}{1000} = \frac{6}{\underset{100}{\cancel{600}}} = \text{gr } \frac{1}{100}$$

Knowing that 0.0006 g is equivalent to gr $\frac{1}{100}$, one can set up the proportion as follows, using grains in place of grams:

grains:grains = tablets:tablets

$$\frac{1}{150} \text{ (gr)}:\frac{1}{100} \text{ (gr)} = x \text{ (tab.)}:1 \text{ (tab.)}$$

$$\frac{1}{100}x = \frac{1}{150}$$

$$x = \frac{1}{150} \div \frac{1}{100}$$

$$x = \frac{1}{150} \times \frac{100}{1} = \frac{\cancel{100}^{2}}{\cancel{150}_{3}} =$$

$$\frac{2}{3} \text{ tab. atropine sulfate, 0.0006 g per tablet}$$

It will be noted that the answer is $\frac{2}{3}$ tab. in both instances.

Exercise

Solve the following problems for correct number of tablets needed, unless indicated otherwise:

1. The physician orders atropine sulfate, 0.4 mg. The dose on hand is gr $\frac{1}{200}$ tablets.
2. The physician orders digitoxin, gr $\frac{1}{300}$. The dose on hand is 0.1 mg tablets.
3. The physician orders thiamine chloride, 200 mg. The dose on hand is gr iss tablets.
4. The physician orders atropine sulfate, gr $\frac{1}{100}$. The dose on hand is 0.0006 g tablets.
5. The physician orders ascorbic acid, gr 3¾. The dose on hand is 0.1 g tablets.
6. The physician orders calcium lactate, 600 mg. The dose on hand is gr x tablets.
7. The physician orders sodium bicarbonate, gr xv. The dose on hand is 0.3 g tablets.
8. The physician orders morphine sulfate, 0.005 g. The dose on hand is gr ¼ tablets.
9. The physician orders Dramamine (dimenhydrinate), 100 mg. The dose on hand is gr ⅚ tablets.
10. The physician orders atropine sulfate, 0.0006 g. The dose on hand is gr $\frac{1}{200}$ tablets.

11. The physician orders phenobarbital, gr ss. The dose on hand is 0.015 g tablets.
12. The physician orders codeine sulfate, gr ss. The dose on hand is 0.015 g tablets.
13. The physician orders codeine sulfate, gr ¼. The dose on hand is 0.06 g tablets.
14. The physician orders atropine sulfate, gr ½₀₀. The dose on hand is 0.4 mg tablets.
15. The physician orders atropine sulfate, 0.6 mg. The dose on hand is gr ½₀₀ tablets.
16. The physician orders codeine, gr i. The dose on hand is 30 mg tablets.
17. The physician orders nicotinic acid, gr iss. The dose on hand is 25 mg tablets.
18. The physician orders morphine sulfate, 0.005 g. The dose on hand is gr ⅙ tablets.
19. The physician orders morphine, gr ¼. The dose on hand is 10 mg tablets.
20. The physician orders Dilaudid, gr ½₃₂. The dose on hand is 4 mg tablets.
21. The physician orders acetylsalicylic acid (aspirin), gr x. The tablets on hand each contain 325 mg.
22. Acetaminophen, 650 mg, is ordered. This is approximately equivalent to how many grains?
23. Amitriptyline hydrochloride is available in 100 mg tablets. One tablet is equivalent to how many grains?
24. If Aldomet, gr 7½, is to be administered, how many 500 mg tablets will be needed for this dose?

27 COMPUTATION OF DOSAGE

When a specific dose is to be given and the label on the bottle reads that a certain amount of drug is dissolved in a certain amount of solution

The physician's order reads that codeine phosphate, gr i (H), is to be given. The label on the bottle reads gr iss in 4 ml (cc). Interpreting the dosage of the label of this bottle, the nurse finds that in every 4 ml (cc) of solution there are gr iss of the drug. This is another way of saying, as was true of solids, that in every tablet there are gr iss; but in this case the solid drug has been dissolved in a solution.

METHOD 1. Establish a proportion using the information on the label as one ratio of the proportion and the desired (prescribed) dose as the other.

Labeling information   **Desired dose**

grains:milliliters = grains:milliliters

$$1\frac{1}{2} \text{ (gr)}:4 \text{ (ml)} = 1 \text{ (gr)}:x \text{ (ml)}$$

$$1\frac{1}{2}x = 4$$

$$x = 4 \div 1\frac{1}{2}$$

$$x = 4 \div \frac{3}{2}$$

$$x = 4 \times \frac{2}{3}$$

$$x = \frac{8}{3} \text{ or } 2\frac{2}{3} \text{ ml (cc) of codeine phosphate, gr iss in 4 ml (cc)}$$

Gr i would be contained in 2⅔ ml (cc) of the solution labeled gr iss in 4 ml (cc). Sometimes the solution reads gr i in 1 ml (cc), gr i in 2 ml (cc), or gr v in a specified number of milliliters (cubic centimeters).

METHOD 2. Establish a proportion, using small is to large as small is to large.

small:large $=$ small:large

grains:grains $=$ milliliters:milliliters

$1 \, (gr):1\frac{1}{2} \, (gr) = x \, (ml):4 \, (ml)$

$$1\frac{1}{2}x = 4$$

$$x = 4 \div \frac{3}{2}$$

$$x = 4 \times \frac{2}{3} = \frac{8}{3}$$

$$x = 2\frac{2}{3} \text{ ml (cc) of codeine phosphate, gr iss in 4 ml (cc)}$$

METHOD 3. Substitute into the following formula:

$$\left(\frac{\text{desired dose}}{\text{available dose (in specified amount of solution)}}\right) \times$$

amount of solution containing the stated available dose $=$

amount of solution needed to give the desired dose

$$\left(\frac{1 \, (gr)}{1\frac{1}{2} \, (gr)}\right) \times 4 \, (ml) = \left(1 \div 1\frac{1}{2}\right) \times 4 = \left(1 \times \frac{2}{3}\right) \times 4 = \frac{8}{3} =$$

$$2\frac{2}{3} \text{ ml (cc) codeine phosphate, gr iss in 4 ml (cc)}$$

Most drugs intended for injection are available in a sterile solution. The label states the amount of drug contained in a specified amount of solution. The practice of supplying the individual dose for injection in a prepackaged form increases control of sterility and helps protect the patient from the use of contaminated solutions. Many drugs intended for injection are supplied in premeasured amounts in sterile disposable syringes or cartridges. Drugs that are not stable in solution form for extended periods are marketed as powders in sterile ampules or vials and are reconstituted as directed by the manufacturer before use. Although hypodermic tablets continue to be marketed, their use for the preparation of a drug dosage that is injected can no longer be justified. The illustration on p. 114 shows examples of syringes that may be used to measure solutions to be injected.

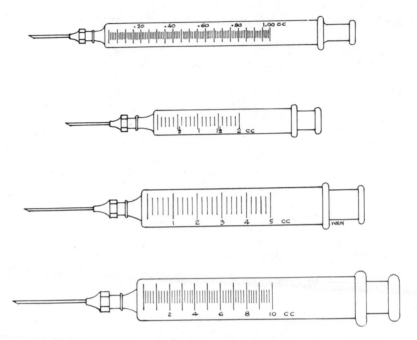

Syringes are used to accurately measure varying amounts of sterile solutions for injection. Uppermost syringe is known as a tuberculin syringe and is graduated in 0.01 ml (cc). It is the syringe of choice for administration of small amounts. Two ml (cc) syringe is one commonly used to give drug subcutaneously (hypodermically), intramuscularly, or intravenously. It is graduated in 0.1 ml. Larger syringes are used when larger volume of drug is to be administered. Note that cc (ml) on all except tuberculin syringe contain markings for each one tenth of cc (ml) in addition to ½ and 1 cc (ml) markings.

Exercise

Solve the following problems for the correct solutions to be administered:

1. The physician's order reads, "Meperidine, 50 mg." The only meperidine available is premeasured in a syringe marked in tenths of a milliliter and labeled, "Meperidine, 75 mg/ml."
2. The physician orders elixir of phenobarbital, gr ss. The dose on hand is in a bottle labeled ʒi = gr ¼.
3. The physician orders sodium salicylate, gr xv. The dose on hand is in a bottle labeled gr xx in 4 ml (cc).
4. The physician orders morphine sulfate, 10 mg (H). The dose on hand is in a solution labeled gr ¼ in 1 ml (cc).
5. The physician orders potassium iodide, gr x. The dose on hand is in a bottle labeled gr xv = ʒi.
6. The physician orders caffeine sodium benzoate, gr ii (H). The dose on hand is an ampule labeled 0.5 g in 2 ml (cc).

114

7. The physician orders histamine phosphate, 0.275 mg (H). The dose on hand is contained in a bottle labeled 0.00275 g in 5 ml (cc).

8. The physician orders sodium bicarbonate, gr xv. The dose on hand is gr v = 4 ml (cc).

9. The physician orders 300,000 units of penicillin (IM). The dose on hand is in solution in a bottle labeled 3,000,000 units per 10 ml (cc).

10. The physician orders that an intravenous needle be flushed with heparin, 50 U. Heparin lock flush solution is available in a disposable syringe labeled, "100 U/ml."

11. The physician orders 0.3 g of potassium iodide. The dose on hand is in a bottle labeled gr xv in 1 ml (cc).

12. The physician orders sodium salicylate, 2 g. The dose on hand is in a solution labeled 0.64 g in 4 ml (cc).

13. The physician orders codeine phosphate, 0.015 g (H). The dose on hand is 0.06 g in 1 ml (cc).

14. The physician orders reserpine, 1.5 mg. The dose on hand is in a solution labeled 0.0025 g in 1 ml (cc).

15. The physician orders morphine sulfate, gr ¼ (H). The dose on hand is in a bottle labeled 0.006 g in ℳxvi.

16. The physician's order is for 25 mg of meperidine (IM). The premeasured dose contains 50 mg/ml.

17. The physician orders Staphcillin, 500 mg. The dose on hand is in a solution labeled 1 g in 1 ml (cc).

18. The physician orders chloral hydrate, gr xv. The dose on hand is in a solution labeled gr x in ʒi.

19. The physician orders meperidine hydrochloride, 50 mg. The dose on hand is in a solution labeled 0.1 g in 1 ml (cc).

20. The physician orders cortisone acetate, 62.5 mg. The dose on hand is in suspension in a container labeled 25 mg in 1 ml (cc).

21. The physician orders streptomycin, 2 g. The dose on hand is in solution labeled 500 mg in 1 ml (cc).

22. The physician orders streptomycin, 0.25 g. The dose on hand is 500 mg in 1 ml (cc).

23. The physician orders methenamine, gr xx. The dose on hand is in a solution labeled 0.64 g in 2 ml (cc).

24. The physician orders penicillin, 150,000 units (IM). The dose on hand is in a bottle labeled 3,000,000 units per 10 ml (cc).

25. The physician orders sodium salicylate, gr xx. The dose on hand is in a solution labeled 0.6 g in 4 ml (cc).

26. The physician orders 2 mg morphine to be given intravenously. The solution available is labeled, "Morphine, 4 mg (1/15 gr)/ml."

28 INSULIN DOSAGE

Regardless of where nursing is practiced, the care of diabetic patients is always a nursing responsibility. It is essential that nurses and patients learn to measure insulin dosages accurately. If the patient receives more insulin than is needed, there is danger that insulin shock will develop, and if the patient receives less insulin than needed, diabetic coma is likely to develop. Both reactions may result in serious, irreversible complications or death if untreated. Nurses who care for patients with diabetes must be able to recognize the symptoms of both hyperglycemia and hypoglycemia.

Different insulin preparations are prescribed depending on the requirements of the patient. Those currently available are:

Fast-acting preparations (act quickly, in about an hour; duration of action varies with preparation)

Insulin injection, U.S.P. (regular insulin)—effects last about 6 hours

Insulin injection, U.S.P. (regular insulin made from zinc-insulin crystals)—effects last about 8 hours

Prompt insulin zinc suspension, U.S.P. (semilente)—effects last about 14 hours

Intermediate-acting preparations (act in about 2 hours; effects last about 24 hours)

Isophane insulin suspension, U.S.P. (NPH insulin, isophane insulin)

Insulin zinc suspension, U.S.P. (lente insulin)

Globin zinc insulin

Long-acting preparations (act in about 7 hours; effects last about 36 hours)

Protamine zinc suspension, U.S.P.

Extended insulin zinc suspension, U.S.P. (ultralente insulin)

The insulin preparations listed are currently available in strengths of

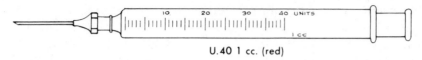

U.40 1 cc. (red)

U-40 insulin syringe. It is used only for U-40 insulin (40 units of insulin in 1 ml [cc]). It is scaled in red.

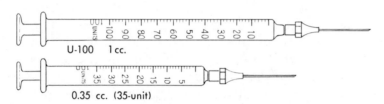

U-100   1 cc.

0.35 cc. (35-unit)

U-100 insulin syringes. Upper syringe is calibrated for measurement of U-100 insulin in amounts up to 100 units or 1 cc. Each calibration represents 2 units of insulin. Lower syringe is used to measure small doses of insulin. Each calibration represents single unit; maximum amount of insulin that can be measured with this syringe is 35 units or 0.35 cc. *Both syringes must be used to measure U-100 insulin only.*

U-40 and U-100.* The names of U-100 insulins are preceded by the word "purified." One fast-acting preparation, Insulin injection, concentrated-purified, is available in 500 U/ml only. This preparation, used in the treatment of insulin-resistant diabetes, must be measured with extreme accuracy because of the potency of the preparation.

Insulin dosage is ordered in units (U). Each unit of insulin provides the patient with the same dose and effect regardless of the number of units of insulin in each milliliter of solution. The strength of the solution does not alter the potency of the unit.

Insulin syringes that are approved for use by the American Diabetes Association are scaled in calibrations for measuring units of insulin. Each syringe is calibrated according to the strength of insulin with which it is to be used. This eliminates any need to calculate dosage. Color-coding of these special syringes corresponds with the color-coding of the insulin preparations. The U-40 syringe has red calibrations and is to be used with U-40 insulin only. Each vial of U-40 insulin is identified with a red cap and red

---

*Manufacture of U-80 insulin has been discontinued in the United States. It is expected that manufacture of U-40 strength of insulin will be discontinued in the future. Knowledge that both the 1 ml and the 2 ml U-80 syringes were calibrated with green scales aids in the recognition of those that have not been destroyed. Clients should be instructed to destroy U-80 syringes in order to prevent serious error in insulin dosage.

lettering on its label. The calibrations of U-100 syringes are either orange or black and are intended for use only with U-100 insulin, which is supplied in vials that have orange caps and black labeling. Either the hub of the needle or the needle protector of the disposable U-100 syringes is also colored orange. These supplies are available from drugstores and pharmaceutical supply houses. Measurement of insulin dosage with any other than the approved insulin syringes increases the potential errors in dosage and thus should be avoided.

Although insulin preparations are available in the strengths of U-40 and U-100, it is the goal of the American Diabetes Association to replace the use of all strengths of insulin and syringes calibrated for their measurement with the use of U-100 insulin and U-100 insulin syringes.* As this goal is achieved, it is expected that the manufacture of insulin in the strength of U-40 and of syringes calibrated in units for the measurement of this concentration will be discontinued.

Changing to U-100 insulin and syringes is expected to reduce errors in dosage, resulting in better management of the diabetic person's health by removing sources of confusion to all who measure doses of insulin. Serious errors in insulin dosage have been related to the measurement of one strength of insulin in a syringe that is calibrated for the measurement of another strength of insulin or is calibrated for the measurement of minims or parts of a milliliter (cubic centimeter). For this reason, other strengths of insulin solutions and syringes calibrated for their measurement should be destroyed when a person or institution converts to the use of U-100 insulin and syringes. Both disposable and reusable syringes are available for the measurement of U-100 insulin.

Adequate education of the patient, the nurse, and the physician is essential. Each must understand the purpose for using a single concentration of insulin and syringes calibrated especially for its measurement. They must understand that the potency of a unit of insulin is always the same regardless of the concentration of the solution. Nearly every diabetic person can be taught to measure dosages accurately using this method.

The following examples illustrate the simple method of measuring insulin dosage with a syringe that is calibrated to match the strength of the insulin solution used:

Problem A. Administer U 25 (H) of regular insulin from a solution labeled U-100 per milliliter.

ANSWER: Withdraw the amount of solution from the U-100 regular insulin preparation to fill a calibrated 0.35 cc U-100 syringe to the U 25 calibration.

---

*Use of U-500 insulin for insulin-resistant diabetes may continue to be an exception to this trend.

Problem B. Administer U 20 (H), using a U-40 syringe and insulin labeled U-40 per milliliter.

ANSWER: Withdraw the amount of solution necessary to fill the U-40 syringe to the U 20 calibration.

Exercise

After working each of the following problems, it is suggested that the correct calibration on the right syringe for measuring the prescribed dose be identified:

1. Give insulin U 5 (H) from U-100 solution, using a U-100 syringe.
2. Give insulin U 8 (H) from U-100 solution, using a U-100 syringe.
3. Give insulin U 16 (H) from U-100 solution, using a U-100 syringe.
4. Give insulin U 45 (H) from U-100 solution, using a U-100 syringe.
5. Give insulin U 20 (H) from U-40 solution, using a syringe with a U-40 scale.
6. Give insulin U 25 (H) from U-40 solution, using a U-40 syringe.
7. Give insulin U 35 (H) from U-100 solution, using a U-100 syringe.
8. Give insulin U 15 (H) from U-40 solution, using a U-40 syringe.
9. Give protamine zinc insulin U 60 (H) from U-100 solution, using a 1-cc, U-100 syringe.
10. Give insulin U 24 (H) from U-100 solution, using a U-100 syringe.
11. Give insulin U 10 (H) from U-100 solution, using a U-100 syringe.
12. Give insulin U 40 (H) from U-40 solution, using a U-40 syringe.
13. Give insulin U 7 (H) from U-100 solution, using a U-100 syringe.
14. Give insulin U 9 (H) from U-40 solution, using a U-40 syringe.
15. Give insulin U 22 (H) from U-100 solution, using a U-100 syringe.
16. Give insulin U 35 (H) from U-40 solution, using a U-40 syringe.
17. Give insulin U 18 (H) from U-40 solution, using a U-40 syringe.
18. Give insulin U 50 (H) from U-100 solution, using a U-100 syringe.
19. Give insulin U 80 (H) from U-100 solution, using a U-100 syringe.
20. Give insulin U 28 (H) from U-40 solution, using a U-40 syringe.
21. Give NPH insulin U 20 (H) from U-100 solution, using a 0.35 cc, U-100 syringe.
22. Give protamine zinc insulin U 60 (H), using U-100 solution and a U-100 syringe.
23. Give insulin U 40 (H) from U-40 solution, using a U-40 syringe.
24. Give insulin, concentrated-purified injection, U 250 from a U-500 solution, using a 2 ml syringe. How many milliliters are needed for the dose?
25. Give insulin, concentrated-purified injection, 400 U from a U-500 solution per 1 ml, using a tuberculin syringe. How many milliliters of solution are needed?

29 COMPUTING A CHILD'S DOSE FROM THE KNOWN ADULT DOSE OF THE DRUG

When prescribed for children, the dosage of many drugs is smaller than the dosage of the same drug for an adult. No one method of computing a child's dose from the adult dose is completely satisfactory. Tables for children's dosage of specific drugs have been developed and published in some pediatric and pharmacology references. Of the many methods for calculating a child's dose, those based on the age of the child are least reliable because factors such as wide variations in the size of a child and the maturity of the child's enzyme systems influence the therapeutic dose.

Regardless of the method used to determine the prescribed dose, observation of the child's response to the dose is critical in assessing whether the dosage needs to be adjusted for the benefit of the individual child. Methods that the nurse might use to determine whether the dose ordered seems reasonable should be recognized as being only guides. The degree of illness may indicate a dosage of certain drugs, such as antibiotics and anticonvulsants, that approximates the dose given to an adult. Computing a child's dose from a total daily adult dose may require dividing the total daily dose into individual doses. This can be done before or after computing the child's dose by dividing the total daily dose by the number of doses to be given daily.

CLARK'S FORMULA

Clark's formula may be used to determine whether the prescribed dose seems reasonable. It is based on the weight of the child and is stated as follows:

$$\frac{\text{weight of the child in pounds}}{150} \times \text{adult dose} = \text{child's dose}$$

EXAMPLE: Using Clark's rule, estimate the dose for a child weighing 30 lb if the adult dose is 2 g.

$$\frac{30}{150} \times 2 = \frac{\cancel{30}}{\cancel{150}} = \frac{\overset{1}{\cancel{3}}}{\underset{5}{\cancel{15}}} \times 2 = \frac{2}{5} \text{ or } 0.4 \text{ g or } 400 \text{ mg}$$

FORMULA BASED ON BODY SURFACE AREA

Methods of determining the child's dose based on body surface area (B.S.A.) are also used. In the absence of nomograms, charts, and tables that list children's dosage, various formulas can be used.

A simple formula may be used to provide a reasonably accurate estimate of body surface area in square meters (m^2) when the child's weight (W.) in kilograms is known. It is considered accurate for patients weighing between 1.5 and 100 kg.

$$\frac{\text{four times child's weight in kilograms} + 7}{\text{child's weight in kilograms} + 90} =$$

body surface area (B.S.A.) in square meters (m^2)

In its abbreviated form, the formula for B.S.A. is stated as follows:

$$\frac{4W. + 7}{W. + 90} = \text{B.S.A. in } m^2$$

EXAMPLE: Determine the body surface area of a child weighing 30 lb.
Step 1: Convert 30 lb to kilograms (there are 2.2 lb in 1 kg):

$$\begin{array}{r}
1\ 3.6 \text{ kg in 30 lb} \\
2.2\overline{)30.0.0} \\
\underline{22} \\
8\ 0 \\
\underline{6\ 6} \\
1\ 4\ 0 \\
\underline{1\ 3\ 2}
\end{array}$$

Step 2: Substitute into formula for body surface area:

$$\frac{(4 \times 13.6) + 7}{13.6 + 90} = \frac{54.4 + 7}{13.6 + 90} = \frac{61.4}{103.6}$$

$$\text{or} \qquad \begin{array}{r} 0.59 \\ 103{,}6.\overline{)61{,}4{,}00} \\ 51\ 8\ 0 \\ 9\ 6\ 00 \\ 9\ 3\ 24 \\ 2\ 76 \end{array}$$

Three steps are used in estimating the child's dose based on body surface area.

EXAMPLE: Calculate the dose for a child weighing 30 lb if the adult dose is 2 g.

Step 1: Convert 30 lb to kilograms, that is, 30 lb = 13.6 kg.

Step 2: Determine the body surface area in square meters. According to the calculation of body surface area in square meters already shown, B.S.A. = 0.59 m^2.

Step 3: Calculate the dosage, using the following formula, which is based on the assumption that an adult weighing 140 lb has a body surface area of 1.7 m^2.

$$\frac{\text{body surface area in square meters}}{1.7} \times$$

$$\text{adult dose} = \text{child's dose}$$

$$\frac{0.59}{1.7} \times 2 \ (g, \text{ the adult dose}) = \text{child's dose}$$

$$\begin{array}{r} 0.34+ \times 2 \ (g.) = 0.68 \text{ g or } 680 \text{ mg} \\ 1{,}7.\overline{)0{,}5.90} \\ 5\ 1 \\ 80 \\ 68 \\ 12 \end{array}$$

From working the same problem with Clark's formula and with the body surface area formula, it is noted that some variations in answers occur; the body surface area is proportionately larger in a small child when compared to the child's weight.

YOUNG'S FORMULA

The formula for Young's rule, which is based on the age of the child in years, follows:

$$\frac{\text{age of the child in years}}{\text{age of the child} + 12} \times \text{adult dose} = \text{child's dose}$$

EXAMPLE: Using Young's rule, estimate the drug dosage for an 8-year-old child if the adult dose is 40 mg.

$$\frac{8}{8 + 12} \times 40 = \frac{8}{\cancel{20}_{1}} \times \frac{\cancel{40}^{2}}{1} = 16 \text{ mg, the estimated dose for an 8-year-old child}$$

Exercises

Calculate the following dosages for children, (a) using Clark's formula and (b) using body surface area:

1. Child weighs 50 lb; adult dose is 30 ml.
2. Child weighs 30 lb; adult dose is 1 ml.
3. Child weighs 75 lb; adult dose is gr x.
4. Child weighs 120 lb; adult dose is 0.1 mg.
5. Child weighs 96 lb; adult dose is 20 µg.
6. Child weighs 102 lb; adult dose is 15 ml.
7. Child weighs 12 lb; adult dose is 40 µg.
8. Child weighs 75 lb; adult dose is ʒiv.
9. Child weighs 20 lb; adult dose is 2 g.
10. Child weighs 80 lb; adult dose is 1000 mg.

Calculate the following dosages for children, using Young's formula:

11. Child is 6 years old; adult dose is 10 mg.
12. Child is 4 years old; adult dose is 2 g.
13. Child is 8 years old; adult dose is gr xx.
14. Child is 9 years old; adult dose is 0.1 g.
15. Child is 6 years old; adult dose is gr x.
16. Child is 8 years old; adult dose is gr x.
17. Child is 10 years old; adult dose is 6 mg.
18. Child is 12 years old; adult dose is 60 mg.
19. Child is 6 years old; adult dose is 0.06 g.
20. Child is 5 years old; adult dose is 4 mg.

30 COMPUTING PROBLEMS RELATED TO INTRAVENOUS SOLUTIONS

Calculating the rate of flow

The nurse is given major responsibility for controlling the rate of flow of intravenous solutions. This requires a basic knowledge of the equipment used and the number of drops per milliliter that can be delivered by the particular equipment in use. The understanding that the number of drops per milliliter of solution varies with the equipment and tubing used makes it imperative that this information be available for accurate computation. For example, one brand of tubing delivers 10 drops per milliliter, whereas the tubing supplied by another manufacturer delivers 15 drops per milliliter; some mechanical pumps deliver 20 drops per milliliter; and special tubing that incorporates a minidropper, which delivers 60 minidrops per milliliter, is available.

In some situations, the containers of intravenous solution are labeled by the pharmacist to indicate the number of drops per minute that must be infused for the solution to be administered within the prescribed time limit. It is often necessary for nurses to calculate and adjust the rate of flow of intravenous solutions for a variety of reasons. These include factors that may change the rate of flow, such as the position of the needle in the vein, the position of the extremity into which the intravenous needle has been placed, the condition of the vein, and interruptions that may occur. Interruptions in the rate of flow may occur as a result of infiltration of the solution into the tissues.

It must be recognized that prescribed amounts of drugs may be administered intravenously. This may be confusing because many drugs are given for a designated time span that is relatively short. Furthermore, the intravenous solution of drug may not be included in the total amount of intravenous fluid that is to be given within the same 24-hour period. If the patient is receiving several doses of drugs in separate containers of 50 or 100 ml of intravenous solution, this may present an additional challenge to the nurse who is regulating the flow of the solutions.

The amount and kind of solution to be given over a specified period of time is prescribed by the physician. The order may state this in a variety of ways, such as the amount of solution to be given within 24 hours, 8 hours, 4 hours, 1 hour, or other time periods. A general principle that is followed in the administration of intravenous fluids is that an even flow rate must be established so that the fluid is delivered at a uniform rate. Failure to maintain a reasonably uniform rate of flow results in the delivery of too much or too little fluid to balance the estimated fluid requirements of the patient. Very rapid infusion may cause serious complications of intravenous therapy, such as circulatory overload leading to congestive heart failure. A rate of flow that is too slow may lead to dehydration and other serious problems.

A formula that may be used to calculate the rate of flow for intravenous solutions follows:*

$$\frac{\text{no. of milliliters of solution} \times \text{no. of drops per mililiter}}{\text{no. of hours for administration} \times 60 \text{ (minutes per hour)}} =$$

$$\text{no. of drops per minute}$$

To solve problems that require calculation of the rate of flow, the known facts are substituted into the formula, and the problem is solved using arithmetic.

EXAMPLE: Give 3 L of intravenous solution during the first 24 hours postoperatively. Information on the container states that there are gtt x per milliliter of solution.

METHOD 1. Substitute directly into the formula:

$$\frac{3000 \text{ (ml of solution)} \times 10 \text{ (gtt per milliliter)}}{24 \text{ (hr)} \times 60 \text{ (min)}} = x \text{ (gtt per minute)}$$

$$\frac{30000 \times 10}{24 \times 60} = \frac{30000}{1440} = \begin{array}{r} 20.8 \\ 1440\overline{)30000.0} \\ \underline{2880} \\ 1200\,0 \\ \underline{1152\,0} \end{array}$$

The decimal is usually rounded off to the whole number. In the above problem rounding off 20.9 tells the nurse that the rate of flow should be approximately 21 drops per minute.

---

*From Dison, N.: Clinical nursing techniques, ed. 4, St. Louis, 1980, The C.V. Mosby Co.

METHOD 2. A similar approach to the problem may be used to determine the amount of solution to be given in a particular period that is less than the total time during which the total amount of solution is to be administered. This method is convenient when several units of solution are ordered or when it is necessary to recalculate the rate of flow. This is an alternate method of working the problem. In the previous example, the total time over which the solution was to be administered was 24 hours, which is divided by 3, the number of liters to be administered. This determines the amount of solution that would be administered in three equal time periods, that is every 8 hours. A proportion may be used to determine the amount of solution that is to be given and would be established as follows:

Amount of solution:time in hours = amount of solution:time in hours

$$3 \text{ (L)}:24 \text{ (hr)} = x \text{ (L)}:8 \text{ (hr)}$$

$$24x = 24$$
$$x = 1 \text{ L per 8-hour period}$$

Following this, the rate of flow can be determined by substituting into the formula previously given or by establishing a second proportion as follows:

total amount of solution in drops	total time of administration in minutes	amount of solution in drops
	:	= : 1 minute

The total amount of solution in drops is found by multiplying the total number of milliliters of solution by the number of drops delivered with the equipment in use. The total time of administration in minutes is determined by multiplying the number of hours by 60, the number of minutes in an hour.

The use of this proportion would be as follows for the previous problem:

$$1000 \text{ (ml of solution)}: \quad 8 \text{ (hr)} \quad = x \text{ (gtt)}:1 \text{ (min)}$$
$$\times \qquad\qquad \times$$
$$10 \text{ (gtt per ml)} \quad 60 \text{ (min per hr)}$$

$$10{,}000 \text{ (ml)}:480 \text{ (min)} = x \text{ (ml)}:1 \text{ (min)}$$

$$480x = 10{,}000$$
$$x = 10{,}000 \div 480 \text{ or } \frac{10{,}000}{480}$$

Either short or long division or cancellation may be used to find x:

$$x = 480\overline{)10000.0}\;\;\; \frac{20.8}{}$$
$$\underline{960}$$
$$400\;0$$
$$\underline{384\;0}$$
$$16\;0$$

or

$$\frac{1000\cancel{0}}{48\cancel{0}} = \frac{125}{6}$$
$$= 20.8$$

x = 20.8 or 21 drops per minute rate of flow in order to administer 1 L, or 1000 ml, solution within 8 hours

Exercise

For each of the following problems, determine the rate of flow per minute unless the problem specifically asks for another unit of measure.

1. Give 1000 ml in 8 hours. There are 10 drops in each milliliter.
2. Give 1 L in 8 hours. There are 15 drops in each milliliter.
3. Give 1000 ml in 8 hours. There are 20 drops in each milliliter.
4. Give 1500 ml in 8 hours. There are 20 drops in each milliliter.
5. Give 1500 ml in 8 hours. There are 15 drops in each milliliter.
6. Give 1 L of solution in 6 hours. There are 15 drops per milliliter of solution.
7. If 1 L is to be given in 8 hours, how many milliliters are to be administered per hour?
8. Give 3500 cc in 24 hours. There are 20 drops per milliliter of solution.
9. Infuse 1 L of solution in 6 hours. There are 15 drops in each milliliter.
10. Give 500 ml in 3 hours using a minidropper that provides 60 minidrops per milliliter.
11. Give 1000 ml of intravenous solution in an hour to test kidney function. There are 10 drops per milliliter.
12. If 1000 ml are to be given in an hour, how many milliliters of solution are to be given in a minute?
13. Give 3000 cc in 24 hours. There are 15 drops in each milliliter.
14. Give 1000 ml in 24 hours. There are 60 drops in each milliliter.
15. Give 3000 ml in 24 hours. There are 20 drops per milliliter.
16. Give 2 L of solution in 24 hours if there are 20 drops per milliliter.
17. Give 2 L of solution in 24 hours if there are 15 drops per milliliter.
18. Give 2 L of solution in 24 hours if there are 10 drops per milliliter.
19. Give 2 L of solution in 24 hours if there are 60 drops in each milliliter.
20. An infant is to be given 10 cc of intravenous solution every hour. A minidropper is used that delivers 60 minidrops per milliliter. How many drops would need to be delivered each minute?

31 COMPUTING PROBLEMS RELATED TO INTRAVENOUS INFUSIONS

Increasing the rate of flow by a specified percent

Theoretically, careful calculation and regulation of the rate of flow ensures that the intravenous solution will be administered over the period that is specified. Realistically, there are many reasons why the rate of flow may be slower than was intended. A major reason for this occurrence is that the intravenous infusion infiltrates the tissue because the needle is displaced. When this happens, it may be necessary to recalculate the rate of flow to deliver the amount of fluids necessary within a given time.

Increasing the rate of flow is accompanied by hazards. For this reason, some hospitals have established guidelines that control the relative rate of increase of flow whenever careful monitoring does not prevent the slowing of the rate of flow. The following is suggested as a method of catching up when the intravenous solution is flowing at a rate that causes the administration of the prescribed volume to be behind schedule. First, assess the patient carefully for signs of circulatory overload and other contraindications for increasing the rate of flow. Common contraindications would include the addition of selected medications to the intravenous solution and the osmolarity of the solution.

If there are no contraindications and the patient is receiving continuous intravenous therapy, the infusion rate may be increased as much as 25% of the basic rate of flow used to deliver the volume of solution over a specific period. The patient is reassessed to determine tolerance to this increased rate of flow. If the patient tolerates the increase well, the rate of flow can be increased by another 25% of the basic rate. This rate of flow is continued until the intravenous solution is on schedule. If these two percentage increases are insufficient to achieve the original schedule, it is necessary to alter the original schedule for infusion. To do this, collaboration with the physician is necessary. A medical order prescribing further increases may be written following the physician's assessment of the patient.

EXAMPLE: If an intravenous infusion schedule that originally demanded that the infusion flow at a rate of 125 ml per hour is behind schedule, one would first determine that 25%, or one fourth, of the prescribed infusion rate of 125 ml is 31 ml. This is done by finding 25% of 125.

$$25\% \times 125$$

or

$$.25 \times 125 = 31.25 \text{ or } 31$$

or

$$\frac{1}{4} \times 125 = \frac{125}{4} \text{ or } 31$$

This amount, 31 in this example, is added to the original base rate to determine the increased rate of flow. By adding 31 (the increase) to 125 (the original rate per hour), the increased rate of flow that can be put into effect is determined.

$$31 + 125 = 156 \text{ ml per hour}$$

Next, the number of drops per minute at which the infusion must flow is determined, as described in Chapter 30.

If a second increase is indicated, the infusion rate is increased another 31 ml per hour, which is 25% of the base rate.

$$31 + 156 = 187 \text{ ml per hour}$$

Exercise

Work each of the following problems in which the rate of flow of intravenous solution is less than is required and agency policy allows a 25% increase of the base rate to occur twice if there are no contraindications. For each problem, state the following answers: (a) the amount in milliliters by which the rate of flow may be increased each hour initially, (b) the total number of milliliters that will be delivered each hour when the initial increase is put into effect, (c) the number of drops per minute of intravenous solution that will be delivered when the initial increase is in effect, (d) the total number of milliliters that may be given hourly if a second increase is indicated, and (e) the number of drops per minute necessary to achieve delivery of the second increase.

1. The intravenous solution was originally scheduled to flow at the rate of 60 ml/hr. There are 60 drops per milliliter.

2. The intravenous solution was originally scheduled to flow at the rate of 50 ml per hour. There are 60 drops in each milliliter.

3. The intravenous solution was originally scheduled to flow at 100 ml per hour. There are 15 drops per milliliter.

4. The intravenous solution was originally scheduled to flow at a rate of 200 cc per hour. There are 10 drops per cubic centimeter.

5. The intravenous solution was originally scheduled to flow at a rate of 3 L in 24 hours. There are 20 drops per milliliter of solution.

6. Each intravenous solution was originally scheduled to flow at a rate of 1 L in 8 hours. There are 60 drops per milliliter.

7. The intravenous solution was originally scheduled at a rate of 2 L in 24 hours. There are 15 drops per milliliter.

8. The intravenous solution was originally scheduled to flow at a rate of 150 ml per hour. There are 15 drops in each milliliter.

9. The intravenous solution was originally scheduled to flow at a rate of 75 ml each hour. There are 60 drops in each milliliter.

10. The intravenous solution was originally scheduled to flow at a rate of 175 ml per hour. There are 20 drops in each milliliter.

32 COMPUTING PROBLEMS RELATED TO INTRAVENOUS INFUSIONS

Determining the amount of drug in a specific amount of solution

Prescribed medications are added to many intravenous solutions. The physician's order may specify that a specific amount of a drug be added to a certain amount of solution that is to be administered over a given period. This controls the amount of drug that is administered so that it is infused at a regular rate. Another method of prescribing intravenous drug therapy is to state that a particular dose of medication is to be placed in a specific amount of solution and that the solution is to be administered at a rate that delivers a fractional amount of the total drug dosage to the patient within a particular time. For example, the order may state that 40 milliequivalents (mEq) of potassium chloride is to be added to 1000 ml of intravenous solution and that it is to be administered at a rate that will deliver 4 mEq of potassium chloride to the patient during each 1-hour period. It is necessary to calculate the rate of flow of the solution needed to deliver the prescribed amount of drug over the time span ordered.

A similar calculation is necessary whenever the amount of drug that has been delivered intravenously in a particular amount of solution needs documentation. This commonly occurs at the end of a 24-hour shift and when infusions are interrupted or discontinued. Such problems can be solved using the proportion method.

Problem A. Give 4 mEq of potassium chloride each hour using 1000 ml of solution that contains 40 mEq of potassium chloride. A proportion may be established as follows:

$$\frac{\text{total amount}}{\text{of drug}} : \frac{\text{total volume}}{\text{of solution}} = \frac{\text{prescribed}}{\text{dose of drug}} : \frac{\text{needed volume}}{\text{of solution}}$$

Substituting into the proportion would be as follows:

$$40 \text{ mEq}:1000 \text{ (ml)} = 4 \text{ mEq}:x \text{ (ml)}$$

$$40x = 1000 \times 4$$
$$40x = 4000$$
$$x = 100 \text{ ml of solution needed to give}$$
$$4 \text{ mEq of potassium chloride}$$

Determination of the rate of flow can be done by substituting into the formula given in Chapter 30. Thus, if 100 ml of solution containing 10 drops per milliliter is to be delivered over a 1-hour (or 60-minute) period, the problem would be worked as follows:

$$\frac{100 \text{ (ml)} \times 10 \text{ (gtt)}}{1(\text{hr}) \times 60 \text{ (min)}} = \frac{1000}{60} = \begin{array}{l}\text{16.6 or 17 drops per minute} \\ \text{would deliver 4 mEq} \\ \text{potassium chloride each} \\ \text{hour from this solution}\end{array}$$

If the solution is to be administered over a period less than 1 hour, the problem may be solved by substituting into the following formula:

$$\frac{\text{total number of drops (ml} \times \text{gtt)}}{\text{total number of minutes}} = \text{drops/minute}$$

EXAMPLE: Give 40 ml of solution over 10 minutes. Each milliliter of solution contains 15 drops.

$$\frac{40 \text{ (ml)} \times 15 \text{ (gtt)}}{10 \text{ (min)}} = \frac{600 \text{ (gtt)}}{10 \text{ (min)}} = 60 \text{ gtt/min}$$

Problem B. An intravenous solution is discontinued after the patient had received approximately 500 ml of the original volume of 1000 ml of solution that contained 80 mEq of potassium chloride. How much potassium chloride did the patient actually receive?

This problem also can be solved using the proportion method.

$$80 \text{ (mEq)}:1000 \text{ (ml)} = x \text{ (mEq)}:500 \text{ (ml)}$$
$$1000x = 80 \times 500$$
$$1000x = 40,000$$
$$x = \frac{40000}{1000} = 40 \text{ mEq of potassium chloride}$$
$$\text{was received by patient}$$

Exercise

Work the following problems:

1. The intravenous solution contains 40 mEq of potassium chloride in 1000 ml of solution. How much potassium chloride will be given when 600 ml of solution has been infused?
2. A 50 ml bag of intravenous solution contains 1.5 million U of ampicillin. How many million units of the drug will have been given when 25 ml of solution has been infused?
3. A 50 ml bag of solution contains 1.5 million U of ampicillin and is to be infused over 20 minutes. (a) What should the rate of flow per minute be if each milliliter contains 15 drops of solution? (b) When the intravenous solution has infused at the correct rate for 12 minutes, how much ampicillin will the patient have received?
4. If an intravenous solution contains 80 mEq of potassium chloride in 1 L of solution, how much potassium chloride will the patient have received when 800 ml of solution remains to be given?
5. The physician writes an order to discontinue intravenous therapy. If the patient was receiving 30 mEq of potassium chloride in 1000 ml of solution and there are approximately 800 ml of solution remaining, how much potassium chloride has the patient received?
6. Regular insulin, 10 U, is added to 1 L of a 5% solution of dextrose in water. This solution is being administered at the rate of 125 ml/hr. (a) At the end of 2 hours, how much regular insulin has been administered? (b) At the end of 6 hours, how much regular insulin has been administered?
7. The intravenous order is as follows: give 1000 ml intravenous solution containing 80 mEq of potassium chloride at 4 mEq of potassium chloride per hour. (a) At what flow rate should the solution be delivered if each milliliter of solution contains 15 drops? (b) At what time would total volume to be administered if the infusion is begun at 8 AM?
8. If 1050 ml of intravenous solution contains 50 g of drug and the solution is to be infused over an 8-hour period, how much drug will the patient receive (a) each hour, and (b) each minute?
9. There is 1 g of drug in 250 ml of intravenous solution. How many drops per minute should the rate of flow be if there are 60 drops in each milliliter and the order is to give 3 mg per minute?
10. Diethylstilbestrol, 1 g in 300 ml of normal saline, is to be administered as follows: 20 gtt for the first 10 minutes, then adjust the rate to give the entire amount over 1 hour. (a) If there are 20 gtt in 1 ml of solution, how much solution will be given in the first 10 minutes? (b) How many milliliters will remain after the first 10 minutes? (c) How many drops per minute must be administered to give the remaining solution within the 1-hour period?

133

33 PREPARING SOLUTIONS

Although many solutions are prepared by pharmaceutical supply houses or the pharmacist, occasions arise in which the nurse is expected to make solutions for irrigations or soaks. For this purpose, either a solid form of the drug (crystals or tablets) or a solution that is stronger than the one being prepared may be used.

The proportion method can be used to solve either of these basic problems. Some explanation is given with examples of each type of problem.

TO MAKE SOLUTION FROM FULL-STRENGTH DRUG (100%)

Problem A. Prepare 1 L of physiologic salt solution. Known facts: the percentage strength of physiologic salt solution is usually accepted as being 0.9%; salt crystals may be considered as 100% or full strength.

METHOD 1. Establish a proportion, using the lesser to the greater strength of solution as one ratio and the lesser to the greater amount of solution as the other ratio needed to form the proportion.

$$\begin{array}{c} \text{lesser} \\ \text{strength} \end{array} : \begin{array}{c} \text{greater} \\ \text{strength} \end{array} = \begin{array}{c} \text{small amount} \\ \text{of solution} \end{array} : \begin{array}{c} \text{total quantity} \\ \text{of solution} \end{array}$$

$$0.9\ (\%) : 100\ (\%) = x\ (\text{ml.}) : 1000\ (\text{ml})$$

$$100x = 0.9 \times 1000$$
$$100x = 900$$
$$x = 900 \div 100 = 9\ \text{g of salt}$$

To make the solution, weigh 9 g of salt, place in a 1000 ml measure, and add water to the 1000 ml calibration.

METHOD 2. Substitute into the following formula:

$$\frac{\text{desired strength (of solution)}}{\text{available strength (of drug)}} \times$$

$$\text{total quantity desired (of finished solution)} =$$

$$\text{amount of drug needed (in its available strength)}$$

$$\frac{0.9(\%)}{100(\%)} \times 1000 \text{ (ml)} = x \text{ (ml or g)}$$

$$\frac{0.9}{1\cancel{00}} \times \frac{10\cancel{00}}{1} = 9.\cancel{0} \text{ g of salt (NaCl)}$$

Problem B. Prepare 500 ml of 4% solution from a pure solution. A pure solution is 100%.

METHOD 1. The proportion would be set up as follows:

$$\text{percent} : \text{percent} = \text{milliliters} : \text{milliliters}$$
$$4(\%) : 100(\%) = x \text{ (ml)} : 500 \text{ (ml)}$$
$$100x = 2000$$
$$x = 2000 \div 100 = 20 \text{ ml of pure solution}$$

Measure 20 ml of the pure solution and add water to make a total of 500 ml of solution.

METHOD 2. Substitute into the formula:

$$\frac{\text{desired strength}}{\text{available strength}} \times \text{total quantity of solution needed} =$$

$$\text{amount of solution (in available strength) needed}$$

This formula may be abbreviated as follows: $\dfrac{D}{A} \times Q = q$

$$\frac{4}{1\cancel{00}} \times 5\cancel{00} = x$$

$$4 \times 5 = 20 \text{ ml of available strength}$$
$$\text{(pure solution) needed}$$

TO MAKE SOLUTION FROM A STOCK SOLUTION

Stock solutions are relatively strong solutions that are diluted to the prescribed weaker strength of solution before using.

Problem A. Prepare 500 ml of 5% boric acid solution from a saturated solution of boric acid. A saturated solution of boric acid is 5.5%.

METHOD 1. Set up a proportion:

percent:percent = milliliters:milliliters
$$5(\%):5.5(\%) = x \ (ml):500 \ (ml)$$
$$5.5x = 2500$$
$$x = 2500 \div 5.5 \text{ or } 454.5 \text{ ml of saturated solution of boric acid}$$

This problem illustrates that *the strength of a saturated solution must be known.*

METHOD 2. Substitute into the formula:

$$\frac{D}{A} \times Q = q$$

$$\frac{5(\%)}{5.5(\%)} \times 500 \ (ml) = q$$
$$2500 \div 5.5 = 454.5 \text{ ml of saturated solution of boric acid}$$

Problem B. Prepare 1 L of 2% cresol solution from a 1:25 solution. To establish a proportion, both strengths must be stated as either percentage or ratio. In the following example, the ratio strength is converted to percentage strength:

$$1:25 = \frac{1}{25} = 25\overline{)1.00} \quad \begin{array}{l} .04 \times 100 = 4\% \end{array}$$
$$\underline{1\ 00}$$

METHOD 1. Set up the proportion:

percent:percent = milliliters:milliliters
$$2(\%):4(\%) = x \ (ml): 1000 \ (ml)$$
$$4x = 2000$$
$$x = 2000 \div 4 = 500 \text{ ml of 4\% (1:25) solution}$$

To make the solution, pour 500 ml of the 1:25 cresol solution into a graduated measure, and add water to make a total of 1000 ml of solution.

METHOD 2. Substitute into the formula:

$$\frac{D}{A} \times Q = q$$

$$\frac{2(\%)}{4(\%)} \times 1000 = q$$

$$\frac{\frac{1}{\cancel{2}}}{\frac{\cancel{4}}{2}} \times 1000 = \frac{1000}{2} = 500 \text{ ml of 4\% (or 1:25) cresol solution}$$

Exercise

Solve the following problems:

1. Make 200 ml of 2% solution of bicarbonate of soda.
2. Prepare 500 ml of a 5% boric acid solution.
3. Prepare 500 ml (cc) of a 1:200 Zephiran solution from a 2% solution.
4. Make 2 L of ⅛% Zephiran solution from a 10% stock solution.
5. Prepare 2.5 L of a 1:20 solution of cresol from a 20% solution.
6. Prepare 1.5 L of a physiologic salt solution.
7. Prepare 1 L of a 5% solution of sodium chloride.
8. Prepare 2 L of a 2.5% boric acid solution.
9. Prepare 1 glassful (240 ml or cc of water) of physiologic salt solution.
10. Prepare 1 L of a ¼% cresol solution from a 1:50 solution.
11. Make 1000 ml (cc) of a 1:1000 solution of potassium permanganate from 0.33 g tablets on hand.
12. Prepare 200 ml of ½% sodium hypochlorite solution from a 5% solution.
13. Prepare 500 ml of 1:500 potassium permanganate solution from a 1:15 solution.
14. Prepare 1000 ml of 2% bichloride of mercury solution, using 0.5 g tablets.
15. Make 500 ml (cc) of 5% sodium bicarbonate solution from 10% stock solution.
16. Prepare a 1:30 solution using ʒi of pure drug.
17. Using ʒii of 3% hydrogen peroxide solution, prepare a 0.5% solution.
18. Prepare 1 L of a 1:1500 solution of potassium permanganate, using a 1:15 solution.
19. Make 500 ml of physiologic salt solution.
20. Prepare 2 gallons of a physiologic salt solution (0.9%).
21. Make 200 ml of 2% solution from 5% boric acid solution.
22. Prepare 0.5 L of a physiologic salt solution.
23. Prepare 1 L of 1:250 potassium permanganate solution from a 1:10 solution.
24. Prepare a 1:100 solution using flʒi of a pure drug.
25. Prepare 500 ml of ½% aluminum acetate from a 5% solution.

ANSWERS TO ARITHMETIC PROBLEMS

Page 5

  I. (1) XIV, (2) XXV, (3) LVII, (4) C, (5) XIII, (6) XLIV, (7) XXXVIII, (8) XIX, (9) V

  II. (1) 110, (2) 6, (3) 46, (4) 29, (5) 17, (6) 4, (7) 25, (8) 91, (9) 1000

  III. (1) 42, (2) 12, (3) 70, (4) 6, (5) 9, (6) 16

  IV. (1) $\frac{4}{5}$, (2) $\frac{1}{50}$, (3) $\frac{1}{4}$, (4) $\frac{3}{4}$, (5) $\frac{2}{5}$, (6) $\frac{1}{5}$

  V. (1) 7, (2) $6\frac{1}{3}$, (3) 2, (4) $17\frac{1}{2}$, (5) $9\frac{5}{8}$, (6) $12\frac{4}{7}$, (7) $11\frac{1}{2}$, (8) $27\frac{1}{5}$, (9) $19\frac{1}{6}$

  VI. (1) $\frac{15}{4}$, (2) $\frac{5}{2}$, (3) $\frac{135}{8}$, (4) $\frac{126}{5}$

  VII. (1) $\frac{3}{4}$, (2) $\frac{9}{20}$, (3) $\frac{3}{10}$, (4) $\frac{6}{7}$

  VIII. (1) $1\frac{7}{24}$, (2) $8\frac{13}{30}$, (3) $1\frac{13}{40}$, (4) $1\frac{73}{90}$

Pages 6 and 7

  IX. (1) $\frac{7}{10}$, (2) $1\frac{7}{8}$, (3) 1, (4) $7\frac{3}{4}$

  X. (1) $\frac{1}{4}$, (2) 27, (3) 35, (4) 13

  XI. (1) One and six tenths, (2) Twenty and seventy-five hundreths, (3) Two hundred and four hundreths, (4) Four hundred fifty and two hundred fifty-one thousandths

  XII. (1) 0.8, (2) 0.75, (3) 0.6, (4) 0.0066 or 0.0067 or 0.007

  XIII. (1) $\frac{1}{100}$, (2) $\frac{25}{100}$ or $\frac{1}{4}$, (3) $\frac{4}{10}$ or $\frac{2}{5}$, (4) $\frac{5}{1000}$ or $\frac{1}{200}$

  XIV. (1) 0.689, (2) 1.565, (3) 1.4278

  XV. (1) 406.739, (2) 126.492, (3) 2062.29

Pages 8 to 10

  XVI. (1) 7.3, (2) 108.54, (3) 8, (4) 183.71

  XVII. (1) 280.08, (2) 51, (3) 728.192, (4) 26.52

  XVIII. (1) $\frac{25}{28}$, (2) $2\frac{2}{3}$, (3) $\frac{8}{81}$, (4) $1\frac{6}{7}$

  XIX. (1) 3.65 plus or 3.66, (2) 6.3, (3) 34.84, (4) 12

  XX. (1) 0.4, (2) 0.078, (3) 0.02, (4) 0.25

  XXI. (1) 0.4, (2) 0.7, (3) 1.8, (4) 4.125

XXII. (1) 6:100 or 3:50, 6%, 0.06; (2) 3:4, 75%, 0.75; (3) 5:1000 or 1:200, 0.5%, 0.005; (4) 1:2, 50%, 0.5

XXIII. (1) 2.4, (2) 2, (3) 3.2, (4) 12

XXIV. (1) 42, (2) 20, (3) 100, (4) 6

Page 11

(1) VIII, (2) X, (3) XV, (4) II, (5) XXIV, (6) XXVI, (7) XXXV, (8) VII, (9) V, (10) XXX, (11) VI, (12) XC, (13) XXIII, (14) XII, (15) IV, (16) XCIII, (17) CC, (18) M, (19) XLVIII, (20) III, (21) L, (22) XIV, (23) XVIII, (24) XIX, (25) LX

Pages 11 and 12

(1) 3, (2) 20, (3) 30, (4) 12, (5) 23, (6) 29, (7) 50, (8) 19, (9) 100, (10) 40, (11) 48, (12) 500, (13) 18, (14) 15, (15) 10, (16) 8, (17) 39, (18) 4, (19) 28, (20) 2000, (21) 6, (22) 24, (23) 90, (24) 1, (25) 16

Page 15

(1)$\frac{3}{16}$, (2) $\frac{1}{3}$, (3) $\frac{3}{4}$, (4) $\frac{1}{4}$, (5) $\frac{1}{4}$, (6) $\frac{5}{6}$, (7) $\frac{1}{2}$, (8) $\frac{3}{8}$, (9) $\frac{2}{3}$, (10) $\frac{4}{5}$, (11) $\frac{1}{3}$, (12) $\frac{1}{8}$,(13) $\frac{1}{2}$, (14) $\frac{1}{4}$, (15) $\frac{1}{4}$, (16) $\frac{1}{2}$, (17) $\frac{1}{12}$, (18) $\frac{1}{4}$, (19) $\frac{1}{5}$, (20) $\frac{1}{2}$, (21) $\frac{2}{5}$, (22) $\frac{7}{8}$, (23) $\frac{3}{5}$,(24) $\frac{1}{2}$, (25) $\frac{1}{4}$

Page 15

(1) 42, (2) 20, (3) 5, (4) 66, (5) 4, (6) 24, (7) 14, (8) 30, (9) 4, (10) 15

Page 16

(1) $1\frac{2}{3}$, (2) $1\frac{1}{4}$, (3) $2\frac{1}{6}$, (4) 8, (5) $17\frac{1}{3}$, (6) $12\frac{3}{4}$, (7) $7\frac{1}{2}$, (8) 3, (9) $3\frac{1}{9}$, (10) 2, (11) 3, (12) $1\frac{5}{6}$, (13) 10, (14) $3\frac{1}{2}$, (15) 4, (16) $5\frac{1}{7}$, (17) $8\frac{1}{2}$, (18) $4\frac{1}{5}$, (19) $4\frac{2}{5}$, (20) $8\frac{2}{5}$, (21) $1\frac{1}{2}$, (22) $1\frac{5}{7}$, (23) $2\frac{1}{3}$, (24) $1\frac{1}{2}$, (25) $6\frac{1}{3}$

Page 17

(1)$\frac{31}{4}$, (2) $\frac{37}{2}$, (3) $\frac{97}{10}$, (4) $\frac{101}{2}$, (5) $\frac{34}{5}$, (6) $\frac{31}{8}$, (7) $\frac{17}{7}$, (8) $\frac{37}{8}$, (9) $\frac{7}{2}$, (10) $\frac{17}{3}$, (11) $\frac{65}{4}$, (12)$\frac{13}{5}$, (13) $\frac{606}{100}$, (14) $\frac{19}{4}$, (15) $\frac{33}{5}$, (16) $\frac{402}{50}$, (17) $\frac{43}{4}$, (18) $\frac{27}{8}$, (19) $\frac{184}{9}$, (20) $\frac{61}{8}$,(21) $\frac{22}{5}$, (22) $\frac{57}{8}$, (23) $\frac{48}{5}$, (24) $\frac{62}{27}$, (25) $\frac{153}{7}$

Pages 18 and 19

(1) $\frac{1}{100}$, (2) $\frac{1}{3}$, (3) $\frac{1}{12}$, (4) $\frac{1}{100}$, (5) $\frac{1}{125}$, (6) $\frac{1}{49}$, (7) $\frac{1}{6}$, (8) $\frac{1}{25}$, (9) $\frac{3}{125}$, (10) $\frac{4}{150}$, (11) $\frac{2}{7}$, (12) $\frac{9}{15}$; (b) (13) $\frac{12}{135}$, (14) $\frac{1}{10}$, (15) $\frac{1}{6}$, (16) $\frac{2}{25}$, (17) $\frac{1}{125}$, (18) $\frac{8}{130}$, (19) $\frac{5}{8}$, (20)

$\frac{9}{80}$, (21) $\frac{3}{50}$, (22) $\frac{5}{7}$, (23) $\frac{1}{150}$, (24) $\frac{4}{10}$; (c) (25) $\frac{8}{9}$, (26) $\frac{5}{6}$, (27) $\frac{5}{9}$, (28) $\frac{4}{5}$, (29) $\frac{7}{9}$, (30) $\frac{7}{30}$, (31) $\frac{4}{5}$, (32) $\frac{7}{8}$, (33) $\frac{4}{25}$, (34) $\frac{3}{10}$, (35) $\frac{3}{50}$

Pages 21 to 23

(1) $1\frac{7}{45}$, (2) $1\frac{4}{9}$, (3) $1\frac{27}{32}$, (4) $1\frac{23}{40}$, (5) $2\frac{9}{32}$, (6) $9\frac{55}{72}$, (7) $73\frac{37}{54}$, (8) $1\frac{1}{9}$, (9) $\frac{9}{32}$, (10) $132\frac{17}{40}$, (11) $1\frac{37}{48}$, (12) $51\frac{1}{2}$, (13) $14\frac{1}{24}$, (14) $6\frac{53}{84}$, (15) $16\frac{41}{96}$, (16) $7\frac{11}{24}$, (17) $47\frac{7}{24}$, (18) $17\frac{13}{24}$, (19) $4\frac{1}{10}$, (20) $60\frac{1}{2}$

Pages 25 and 26

(1) $\frac{1}{20}$, (2) $\frac{1}{27}$, (3) $\frac{1}{5}$, (4) $\frac{7}{16}$, (5) 0, (6) $\frac{3}{10}$, (7) $\frac{1}{4}$, (8) $2\frac{1}{10}$, (9) $7\frac{1}{2}$, (10) $\frac{23}{24}$, (11) $\frac{3}{4}$, (12) $4\frac{1}{8}$, (13) $10\frac{2}{5}$, (14) $12\frac{2}{3}$, (15) $168\frac{5}{8}$, (16) $10\frac{1}{4}$, (17) $58\frac{3}{5}$, (18) $10\frac{5}{12}$, (19) $28\frac{1}{2}$, (20) $47\frac{1}{12}$, (21) $44\frac{9}{10}$, (22) $157\frac{9}{14}$, (23) $54\frac{29}{60}$, (24) $95\frac{3}{50}$, (25) $38\frac{1}{2}$

Page 28

(1) $\frac{7}{16}$, (2) $\frac{4}{11}$, (3) $\frac{1}{3}$, (4) $\frac{1}{4}$, (5) $\frac{2}{5}$, (6) $\frac{1}{6}$, (7) $\frac{5}{48}$, (8) $\frac{1}{6}$, (9) $\frac{20}{27}$, (10) $\frac{16}{45}$, (11) $\frac{3}{80}$, (12) $\frac{7}{250}$, (13) $\frac{6}{25}$, (14) $4\frac{71}{96}$, (15) $14\frac{7}{8}$, (16) $6\frac{3}{32}$, (17) $30\frac{1}{16}$, (18) $72\frac{4}{25}$, (19) $7\frac{2}{9}$, (20) 99, (21) $177\frac{47}{64}$, (22) $176\frac{1}{24}$, (23) $5\frac{179}{392}$, (24) $4748\frac{5}{8}$, (25) $812\frac{11}{24}$

Pages 30 and 31

(1) $1\frac{1}{3}$, (2) $\frac{9}{20}$, (3) $\frac{1}{70}$, (4) $\frac{3}{8}$, (5) $\frac{2}{3}$, (6) $\frac{2}{3}$, (7) 2, (8) $\frac{5}{12}$, (9) $\frac{6}{7}$, (10) $\frac{25}{93}$, (11) 2, (12) $1\frac{1}{3}$, (13) $1\frac{41}{85}$, (14) $\frac{5}{16}$, (15) $\frac{1}{3}$, (16) $\frac{1}{30}$, (17) $5\frac{1}{3}$, (18) $1162\frac{1}{2}$, (19) $9\frac{3}{7}$, (20) $3\frac{65}{93}$, (21) $51\frac{2}{3}$, (22) $68\frac{4}{7}$, (23) $2\frac{12}{65}$, (24) 4, (25) $2\frac{33}{74}$

Pages 32 and 33

(1) eight and thirty-five hundredths, (2) six hundredths, (3) twenty-three and seven tenths, (4) one and twenty-three hundredths, (5) three and eight hundred twenty-one thousandths, (6) nine tenths, (7) eight tenths, (8) nine thousandths, (9) two and five tenths, (10) four and six hundredths, (11) one hundreth, (12) fifteen thousandths

Pages 33 and 34 *(Answers rounded to thousandths)*

(1) 0.04, (2) 0.06, (3) 0.625, (4) 0.4, (5) 0.02, (6) 0.75, (7) 0.5, (8) 0.1, (9) 0.857, (10) 0.08, (11) 0.375, (12) 0.12, (13) 0.9, (14) 0.556, (15) 0.8, (16) 0.6, (17) 0.02, (18) 0.007, (19) 0.417, (20) 0.75, (21) 0.004, (22) 0.005, (23) 0.7, (24) 0.833, (25) 0.2

Page 34

(1) $\frac{1}{2}$, (2) $\frac{18}{25}$, (3) $\frac{2}{5}$, (4) $\frac{13}{200}$, (5) $\frac{17}{20}$, (6) $\frac{3}{25}$, (7) $1\frac{1}{2}$, (8) $\frac{3}{8}$, (9) $\frac{3}{50}$, (10) $\frac{1}{5}$, (11) $\frac{1}{1000}$, (12) $\frac{1}{25}$, (13) $\frac{13}{20}$, (14) $\frac{3}{5000}$, (15) $\frac{3}{5}$, (16) $\frac{7}{25}$, (17) $\frac{1}{2000}$, (18) $\frac{1}{10}$, (19) $2\frac{4}{5}$, (20) $\frac{3}{4}$, (21) $\frac{1}{4}$, (22) $\frac{1}{25,000}$, (23) $\frac{9}{10}$, (24) $\frac{3}{20}$, (25) $5\frac{1}{5}$

Pages 35 and 36

(1) 19.7, (2) 66.303, (3) 30.4, (4) 59.3, (5) 7.305, (6) 40.5, (7) 5.314, (8) 11.275, (9) 48.186, (10) 22.502, (11) 55.165, (12) 26.458, (13) 32.755, (14) 313.426, (15) 87.477, (16) 0.265, (17) 65.841, (18) 91.843, (19) 15.609, (20) 29.1101, (21) 935.267, (22) 301.747, (23) 32.974, (24) 64.651, (25) 174.937

Pages 37 and 38

(1) 3.13, (2) 3.284, (3) 1.3, (4) 45.1, (5) 18.21, (6) 26.75, (7) 3.3, (8) 2.72, (9) 3.11, (10) 2.875, (11) 33.8, (12) 17.64, (13) 27.5, (14) 5.12, (15) 15.87, (16) 15.2, (17) 3.89, (18) 91.196, (19) 129.71, (20) 88.305, (21) 80.78, (22) 3.13, (23) 0.4, (24) 7.83, (25) 253.418

Pages 40 and 41

(1) 5.6, (2) 13.5, (3) 0.775, (4) 13.05, (5) 318.5, (6) 64.12, (7) 29.73996, (8) 302.706, (9) 613.534, (10) 0.001286, (11) 61.6, (12) 76.95, (13) 332.94, (14) 0.04588, (15) 3.645, (16) 0.0054, (17) 2458.8, (18) 320, (19) 60.72, (20) 33.074, (21) 1.912, (22) 4, (23) 84.129, (24) 13.5, (25) 787.449

Pages 42 and 43 *(Answers rounded to thousandths)*

(1) 140, (2) 0.93, (3) 2.592, (4) 0.04, (5) 5500, (6) 0.12, (7) 0.013, (8) 4, (9) 12.8, (10) 9.1, (11) 2, (12) 1.5, (13) 2.574, (14) 4.022, (15) 10, (16) 0.001, (17) 0.02, (18) 4.306, (19) 0.42, (20) 1.8, (21) 0.957, (22) 5, (23) 9, (24) 0.334, (25) 40.262

Pages 43 and 44

(1) 0.6, (2) 0.12, (3) 0.9, (4) 2.48, (5) 0.840, (6) 0.850, (7) 0.2, (8) 0.725, (9) 0.9, (10) 0.04, (11) 0.06, (12) 0.750, (13) 0.45, (14) 0.325, (15) 0.025, (16) 0.003, (17) 0.090, (18) 0.04, (19) 0.05, (20) 0.45, (21) 0.025, (22) 0.001, (23) 0.064, (24) 0.7, (25) 0.04

Pages 45 and 46

Decimals: (1) 0.08, (2) 0.15, (3) 0.9, (4) 0.2, (5) 0.0005, (6) 0.67, (7) 0.1, (8) 0.98, (9) 0.4, (10) 0.00005, (11) 0.0006, (12) 0.12, (13) .088, (14) 0.092

Fractions: (1) $\frac{2}{25}$, (2) $\frac{3}{20}$, (3) $\frac{9}{10}$, (4) $\frac{1}{5}$, (5) $\frac{1}{2000}$, (6) $\frac{67}{100}$, (7) $\frac{1}{10}$, (8) $\frac{49}{50}$, (9) $\frac{2}{5}$, (10) $\frac{1}{20,000}$, (11) $\frac{3}{5000}$, (12) $\frac{3}{25}$, (13) $\frac{11}{125}$, (14) $\frac{23}{250}$

Percents: (1) 45%, (2) 4.3% or $4\frac{3}{10}$%, (3) 25%, (4) 6.5% or $6\frac{1}{2}$%, (5) 125.6%

or $125\frac{3}{5}\%$, (6) 12.5% or $12\frac{1}{2}\%$, (7) 220%, (8) 248%, (9) 75%, (10) 7.5% or

$7\frac{1}{2}\%$, (11) 1.5% or $1\frac{1}{2}\%$, (12) 16%, (13) 1575%, (14) 10%, (15) 80%, (16)

68%, (17) 12%, (18) 57%, (19) 45.5% or $45\frac{1}{2}\%$, (20) 0.8% or $\frac{4}{5}\%$, (21) 15%,

(22) 50%, (23) 0.9% or $\frac{9}{10}\%$ (24) 1830%, (25) 912%

Pages 47 and 48

(1) $\frac{2}{25}$, (2) $\frac{2}{3}$, (3) $\frac{1}{5}$, (4) $3\frac{19}{50}$, (5) $16\frac{7}{9}$, (6) 44, (7) $\frac{1}{2}$, (8) $1\frac{35}{57}$, (9) $3\frac{9}{10}$, (10) 1, (11) $2\frac{17}{44}$,

(12) $3\frac{10}{11}$, (13) 0.46, (14) 4.32, (15) 6.2328, (16) 61.3, (17) 3.7, (18) 1.08, (19) 2,

(20) 4.875, (21) 2, (22) 8.25, (23) 150.7, (24) 20, (25) 1.6

Pages 50 and 51

(1) 1:2, (2) 2:3, (3) 4:5, (4) 3:7, (5) 8:9, (6) 45:87, (7) 5:9, (8) 3:8, (9) 1:2,
(10) 5:6, (11) 2:5, (12) 1:3, (13) 5:6, (14) 9:25, (15) 1:2, (16) 4:5, (17) 1:100,
(18) 21:50, (19) 13:20, (20) 41:50, (21) 2:5, (22) 3:100, (23) 1:4, (24) 9:20,
(25) 1:1000, (26) 1:100, (27) 1:10, (28) 7:1000, (29) 1:5000, (30) 1:200, (31)

1:125, (32) 3:5000, (33) 1:20, (34) 17:100, (35) $33\frac{1}{3}$:100 or 1:3, (36) 1:50,

(37) 9:1000, (38) 4:1000

Page 53 *(Answers rounded to hundredths)*

(1) 8, (2) 1000, (3) 28, (4) 100, (5) $\frac{2}{3}$, (6) 1250, (7) 165, (8) 3.2 or $3\frac{1}{5}$, (9) 6, (10)

40, (11) 2, (12) 40, (13) 42, (14) 4.8 or $4\frac{4}{5}$, (15) 0.8 or $\frac{4}{5}$, (16) 34.29 or $34\frac{2}{7}$, (17)

2.25 or $2\frac{1}{4}$, (18) 0.5 or $\frac{1}{2}$, (19) 0.8, (20) 1.5 or $1\frac{1}{2}$, (21) 20, (22) 28, (23) 15, (24)

7.5 or $7\frac{1}{2}$, (25) 1

Pages 59 and 60

Weight: (1) 0.0001, (2) 2000, (3) 500, (4) 300, (5) 15, (6) 2.5, (7) 0.008, (8) 0.01, 9)
0.005, (10) 0.03, (11) 0.001, (12) 0.0005, (13) 1200, (14) 50,000, (15) 4,
(16) 5, (17) 0.015, (18) 2500, (19) 0.06, (20) 0.0002, (21) 1000, (22)
0.00004, (23) 0.4, (24) 0.05, (25) 0.2, (26) 0.05, (27) 0.025, (28) 8, (29)
20,000, (30) 6.5

Volume: (1) 14, (2) 1000, (3) 500, (4) 0.5, (5) 1000, (6) 20, (7) 5, (8) 0.002, (9) 4,
(10) 0.25, (11) 0.02, (12) 100, (13) 400, (14) 750, (15) 0.2, (16) 0.005, (17)
850, (18) 0.03, (19) 0.6, (20) 150

Pages 63 and 64

Volume: (1) 8, (2) 240, (3) 60, (4) 0.5 or $\frac{1}{2}$, (5) 32, (6) $\frac{1}{4}$ or 0.25, (7) $\frac{1}{8}$, (8) 8, (9) 3,

(10) 480, (11) $\frac{1}{2}$ or 0.5, (12) 30, (13) 4, (14) 2, (15) $\frac{1}{2}$ or 0.5, (16) 16, (17) 64, (18) $\frac{1}{2}$ or 0.5, (19) 1

Pages 63, 64, and 65

Weight: (1) 8, (2) $\frac{1}{4}$ or 0.25, (3) 24 (32 avoirdupois), (4) $\frac{1}{2}$ or 0.5, (5) 60, (6) 16, (7) $\frac{1}{4}$ or 0.25, (8) 32, (9) $\frac{3}{4}$ or 0.75, (10) 6, (11) $\frac{1}{2}$ or 0.5 $\left(\frac{3}{8}\right.$ or 0.375 avoirdupois$\left.\right)$, (12) (13) 120, (14) $\frac{1}{2}$ or 0.5, (15) 480 or 450, (16) 4, (17) 30

Symbols and abbreviations: (1) ℥, (2) ℨ, (3) C, or gal, (4) O or pt, (5) ℳ, (6) lb, (7) gr, (8) qt

Units of measure: (1) ounce, (2) gallon, (3) pint, (4) minim, (5) grain, (6) pound, (7) quart, (8) liter, (9) dram, (10) pint, (11) fluidounce, (12) fluidram

Page 68

(1) 10, (2) 3000, (3) 16, (4) 1.5, (5) 100, (6) 75, (7) 500, (8) 50, (9) 250, (10) 320, (11) 40, (12) 4.8, (13) 640, (14) 2000, (15) 1500, (16) 0.0005, (17) 0.008, (18) 0.012, (19) 0.05, (20) 0.34, (21) 0.032, (22) 0.01, (23) 0.06, (24) 2.2, (25) 0.2, (26) 0.12, (27) 0.016, (28) 0.027, (29) 0.008, (30) 0.25

Page 69* *(Answers rounded to hundredths)*

(1) 60, (2) 54.54, (3) 16, (4) 4, (5) 1000, (6) 45, (7) 2, (8) 1 (9) 30, (10) 8000, (11) 900 or 1000, (12) 3.409 or 3.41, (13) 300, $333\frac{1}{3}$, or 333.33, (14) 600, $666\frac{2}{3}$, or 666.67, (15) 81 or 81.82, (16) 3150 or 3181.82, (17) 225 or 227.27, (18) 2.25 or 2.27, (19) 1200, (20) 33.75 or 34.09, (21) $22\frac{1}{2}$ or 22.5, (22) 2, (23) $\frac{1}{2}$ or 0.5, (24) 1, (25) $\frac{1}{2}$ or 0.5, (26) 22.5, (27) 1.5 or 1.7, (28) 30, (29) $7\frac{1}{2}$, 7.5, or 8.33, (30) 90 or 100, (31) 30 or 33.33, (32) $\frac{1}{4}$, $\frac{4}{15}$ or 0.27, (33) $\frac{1}{2}$, $\frac{8}{15}$, 0.53, $\frac{12}{25}$, or 0.48, (34) $\frac{3}{8}$, $\frac{2}{5}$ or 0.4, (35) 165 or 166.67, (36) 12.1 or 12.22, (37) 0.67 or $\frac{2}{3}$, (38) 22, (39) 17.6, (40) 77 or 77.78

Page 72

(1) viii, (2) 4, (3) 2, (4) 30 or 33.33, (5) 1 or $\frac{4}{5}$, (6) 4, (7) 1, (8) 2, (9) 60 or 66.67, (10) 1, (11) 4, (12) 45 or 50, (13) 15, (14) 8, (15) 30, (16) 1, (17) 2, (18) 2, (19) 15, (20) 0.72 or 0.9, (21) 20, (22) 4, (23) 1.5 or 1.2, (24) 180, (25) $\frac{2}{3}$, $0.66\frac{2}{3}$, $\frac{5}{8}$, or 0.425

---

*Variations in answers occur and are dependent on the approach taken in converting from one system of measures to another.

(1) 2000, (2) 100, (3) 10, (4) 55, (5) 280, (6) 0.45, (7) 80, (8) 172.5, (9) 18, (10) 4, (11) 1, (12) 200, (13) 3, (14) 5, (15) 450, (16) 572.5, (17) (a) 2.5, (b) 2, (18) 20, (19) decrease, (20) 5

(1) 50, (2) 2.7, (3) 4, (4) 135, (5) 0.56, (6) 118.2, (7) 21, (8) 2.67 or $2\frac{2}{3}$, (9) 5, (10) 375, (11) 4, (12) 2.7, (13) 30, (14) 4.4, (15) 10, (16) 1, (17) 42.5, (18) 22, (19) 15, (20) 236.4, (21) (a) 185, (b) 1.85 or 1.89, (22) 162.5, (23) 52.5, (24) 2.5, (25) 3.75, (26) 30, (27) (a) increasing, (b) 82.5, (28) 6.09 or 6, (29) 66 or 65.67, (30) 800, (31) 88, (32) 155, (33) (a) 4.375, (b) 7.5, (c) 3.125 or $3\frac{1}{8}$, (34) 3.5, (35) 3.75, (36) 6.25, (37) 28

(1) $36\frac{2}{9}$ or 36.222, (2) $38\frac{5}{9}$ or 38.56, (3) $38\frac{1}{9}$ or 38.111, (4) $37\frac{1}{9}$ or 37.111, (5) 42.2 or $42\frac{2}{9}$, (6) 34.44 or $34\frac{4}{9}$, (7) 38.89 or $38\frac{8}{9}$, (8) 36.66 or $36\frac{2}{3}$, (9) 37.56 or $37\frac{5}{9}$, (10) 39.89 or $39\frac{8}{9}$, (11) 96.8, (12) 103.28, (13) 100.04, (14) 104, (15) 100.76 or 100.8, (16) 208.4, (17) $98\frac{24}{25}$ or 98.96, (18) 122, (19) 185, (20) $98\frac{6}{25}$ or 98.24 or 98.24

(1) (a) 1.5 ml (cc), (b) intramuscularly; (2) (a) 1 tab. neomycin labeled 0.5 g, (b) orally; (3) (a) 1, (b) subcutaneously; (4) (a) 1 tab. phenobarbital, 30 mg, (b) four times each day, (c) according to table 3, 9—1—4—7; (5) (a) 1 cap. Darvon, plain, 32 mg, (b) every 6 hours; (6) (a) 1 cap, Darvon Compound-65, (b) 3 hours, (c) if needed, as necessary; (7) (a) 1 ml, (b) intravenous, (c) immediately, (d) no, (e) units, (f) ask your employer or instructor; (8) (a) 2 drams, (b) every other hour (that is, every 2 hours), (c) on the alternate hours (that is, on the hours when the drug is not given); (9) (a) 1 ounce, (b) $\frac{1}{2}$ hour before meals; (10) (a) liquid, (b) 10 drops, (c) three times a day; (11) (a) 10 grains, (b) 10 grains; (12) (a) rectally, (b) do not repeat this dose, (c) $7\frac{1}{2}$ grains; (13) (a) drops, (b) right, (c) twice daily, (d) o.u.; (14) Antibiotic preparations are given at equally spaced time intervals to keep the blood level constant; this prevents organisms from developing resistance to antibiotic drugs and assists in the inhibition of their growth or the killing of the organisms. She can adjust the time she takes the first capsule each day to fit her schedule, as long as she maintains the necessary equal time intervals throughout the day. (15) (a) Taking the drug at the time intervals prescribed is necessary to maintain the right amount of drug in the blood for controlling her symptoms. The physician will schedule blood tests

periodically; these tests will enable the physician to regulate the dose of the drug. (b) Planning with Susan allows her to determine the best times for her to take the medication within her usual pattern of daily activities. For example, if she usually arises at 8 AM, this would be a natural time for her to take her first dose of medication. However, if she prefers to take the second dose of medication at 7 PM and usually sleeps until 11 AM, she may decide that she prefers to take the first dose of medication at 7 AM because she finds it easy to go back to sleep. Multiple alternatives are possible; the important consideration is finding a schedule that is compatible with the requirements of the prescribed drug therapy and the preferences of the patient. (c) To progress from total dependence on the nurse to independence through self-medication, a plan would be devised into which Susan has input. At first, the nurse might remind Susan that it is time to take her medication and ask that she come to the nurse's station to prepare and take each dose; before her dismissal, Susan would be asked to demonstrate complete responsibility for her own drug therapy. The use of checklists and multiple opportunities to practice this responsibility allows for corrective teaching as well as for the development of self-confidence and good habits. (d) The nurse usually takes this responsibility. (16) Considerations might include always making certain that she carries an adequate supply of medication with her when she plans to be away from home, carrying a copy of her prescription with her, telephoning her physician, or asking a physician in private practice or who is contacted through an emergency service to contact her physician so she may obtain an emergency supply of medication. (17) One alternative is that she might consider taking the drug only after eating, if she has previously been taking the drug without eating. Another alternative is to change the time schedule so that two capsules are taken each time, instead of three capsules. With the physician's approval, she might follow a time schedule that approximates 8-hour intervals. (18) One plan might be as follows: 7:30 AM—Nefedipine, Isordil, Tenormin, Trans-derm 5, and Colace; 1 PM—Nefedipine, Isordil; 5 PM—Isordil; 10 PM— Nefedipine, Isordil. Other variations could be planned according to the time the patient usually awakens and retires. (19) (a) one, (b) Darvon N-100, (c) every 3 to 4 hours. (20) If the medication wrapper has not been opened.

Pages 101 and 102

(1) 2, (2) 2, (3) $\frac{1}{3}$, (4) 2, (5) 3, (6) 2, (7) 2, (8) 2, (9) 2, (10) $\frac{1}{2}$, (11) $\frac{1}{2}$, (12) $1\frac{1}{2}$, (13) 2, (14) 3, (15) 2, (16) 2, (17) 1, (18) 8, (19) 2, (20) 4, (21) 3, (22) 12, (23) 3, (24) 8, (25) 4

Pages 105 to 107

(1) 2, (2) 2, (3) $\frac{2}{3}$, (4) 0.5, (5) $\frac{2}{3}$, (6) $\frac{2}{3}$, (7) 4, (8) $\frac{1}{3}$, (9) 2, (10) 5, (11) 0.25, (12) $1\frac{1}{2}$, (13) $\frac{1}{3}$, (14) 2, (15) $\frac{3}{4}$, (16) 4, (17) 3, (18) 0.5, (19) 4, (20) $\frac{1}{3}$, (21) 2, (22) $1\frac{1}{2}$, (23) $\frac{5}{6}$, (24) 4, (25) 3, (26) 0.5, (27) $\frac{2}{3}$, (28) $\frac{2}{3}$, (29) 4, (30) 3

Pages 110 and 111*

(1) $1\frac{1}{3}$ or $1\frac{1}{5}$, (2) 2, (3) 2 or $2\frac{2}{9}$, (4) 1 or 1.1, (5) $2\frac{1}{2}$ or $2\frac{1}{4}$, (6) 1 or 0.9, (7) 3, 3.1, or 3.3, (8) $\frac{1}{3}$, $\frac{3}{10}$, 0.32, or $\frac{8}{25}$, (9) 2 or $1\frac{4}{5}$, (10) 2 or $1\frac{4}{5}$, (11) 2 or $2\frac{2}{9}$, (12) 2 or $2\frac{2}{9}$, (13) $\frac{1}{4}$ or $\frac{5}{18}$, (14) $\frac{3}{4}$ or $\frac{5}{6}$, (15) 1, (16) 2 or $2\frac{2}{9}$, (17) 3.67, $3\frac{3}{5}$, or 4, (18) $\frac{1}{2}$ or $\frac{9}{20}$, (19) $1\frac{1}{2}$ or $1\frac{2}{3}$, (20) $\frac{1}{2}$ or $\frac{15}{32}$, (21) 2.05 or 2, (22) $10\frac{5}{6}$ gr, (23) $1\frac{2}{3}$ gr, (24) $\frac{9}{10}$

Pages 114 and 115

(1) 6.7 tenths of 1 ml or $\frac{2}{3}$ ml (cc), (2) 3ii, (3) 3 ml (cc), (4) $\frac{2}{3}$ ml (cc), (5) $3\frac{2}{3}$, (6) $\frac{8}{15}$, $\frac{12}{25}$, or .48 ml (cc), (7) 0.5 ml (cc), (8) 12 ml (cc), (9) 1 ml (cc), (10) $\frac{1}{2}$ ml (cc), (11) 0.3 ml (cc), (12) 12.4 ml (cc), (13) 0.25 ml (cc), (14) 0.6 ml (cc), (15) ℳ40, $41\frac{2}{3}$, or $37\frac{1}{2}$, (16) $\frac{1}{2}$ ml (cc), (17) 0.5 ml (cc), (18) f𝔷iss, (19) 0.5 ml (cc), (20) 2.5 ml (cc), (21) 4 ml (cc), (22) 0.5 ml (cc), (23) 3.75, $3\frac{3}{4}$, or $4\frac{1}{6}$ ml (cc), (24) 0.5 ml (cc), (25) 8 ml (cc), (26) $\frac{1}{2}$ ml (cc)

Page 119

(1) U 5, (2) U 8, (3) U 16, (4) U 45, (5) U 20, (6) U 25, (7) U 35, (8) U 15, (9) U 60, (10) U 24, (11) U 10, (12) U 40 or 1 cc, (13) U 7, (14) U 9, (15) U 22, (16) U 35, (17) U 18, (18) U 50, (19) U 80, (20) U 28, (21) U 20, (22) U 60, (23) U 40 or 1 cc, (24) 0.5 ml (cc), (25) 0.8 ml (cc)

Page 123

(1) (a) 10 ml, (b) 15 or 15.3 ml; (2) (a) 0.2 or $\frac{1}{5}$ ml, (b) 0.34 or 0.35 ml; (3) (a) gr v, (b) 6.76, 6.8, or 6.82 grains; (4) (a) 0.08 or $\frac{2}{25}$ mg, (b) 0.089 or 0.091 mg; (5) (a) 12.8 or $12\frac{4}{5}$ µg, (b) 15.8 or 16 µg; (6) (a) 10.2 or $10\frac{1}{5}$ ml, (b) 12.3 or 12.45 ml; (7) (a) 3.2 or $3\frac{1}{5}$ µg, (b) 7, 7.05, 7.1, or 7.2 µg; (8) (a) 𝔷ii, (b) 2.7 or 2.72 drams; (9) (a) $\frac{4}{15}$ or 0.27 g, (b) 0.52 or 0.56 g; (10) (a) $533\frac{1}{3}$, (b) 700, 705.88, or 710 mg; (11) $3\frac{1}{3}$ mg; (12) $\frac{1}{2}$ g; (13) gr viii; (14) 0.04 or $\frac{3}{70}$ g; (15) gr $3\frac{1}{3}$ or 3.33; (16) gr iv; (17) 2.72 or $2\frac{8}{11}$ mg; (18) 30 mg; (19) 0.02 g; (20) 1.176 or 1.18 mg

---

*Variations in answers occur and are dependent on the approach taken in converting from one system to another.

Page 127

(1) 20.83, $20\frac{5}{6}$, or 21, (2) 31.25, $31\frac{1}{4}$, or 31, (3) 41.66, 41.7, $41\frac{2}{3}$, or 42, (4) 62.5, $62\frac{1}{2}$, or 63, (5) 46.87, 46.9, $46\frac{7}{8}$, or 47, (6) 41.66, $41\frac{2}{3}$, or 42, (7) 125, (8) 48.6, $48\frac{11}{48}$, or 49, (9) 41.66, $41\frac{2}{3}$, or 42, (10) 166.66, $166\frac{2}{3}$, or 167, (11) 166.66, $166\frac{2}{3}$, or 167, (12) 16.66, $16\frac{2}{3}$, or 17, (13) 31.25, $31\frac{1}{4}$, or 31, (14) 41.66, 41.7, $41\frac{2}{3}$, or 42, (15) 41.66, 41.67, $41\frac{2}{3}$, or 42, (16) 27.77, $27\frac{7}{9}$, or 28, (17) 20.83, $20\frac{5}{6}$, or 21, (18) 13.88, $13\frac{8}{9}$, or 14, (19) 83.3, $83\frac{1}{3}$, or 83, (20) 10

Pages 129 and 130

(1) (a) 15, (b) 75, (c) 75, (d) 90, (e) 90; (2) (a) 12.5, (b) 62.5, or $62\frac{1}{2}$, (c) 62.5 or $62\frac{1}{2}$, (d) 75, (e) 75; (3) (a) 25, (b) 125, (c) 31.25, $31\frac{1}{4}$, or 31, (d) 150, (e) 37.5, $37\frac{1}{2}$, or 38; (4) (a) 50, (b) 250, (c) 41.66, $41\frac{2}{3}$, or 42, (d) 300, (e) 50; (5) (a) 31.25, $31\frac{1}{4}$, or 31, (b) 156 or $156\frac{1}{4}$, (c) 52, (d) 187, 187.5, or 188, (e) 62.5, $62\frac{1}{2}$, 62.6, $62\frac{2}{5}$, or 63; (6) (a) 31.25, (b) 156.25 or $156\frac{1}{4}$, (c) 156 or 156.25, (d) 187.5 or 187, (e) 187.25 or 188; (7) (a) 20.8, $20\frac{5}{6}$, or 21, (b) $104\frac{1}{6}$, 104.13, or 104, (c) 26, (d) 124.9 or 125, (e) 31.25 or 31; (8) 37.5 or $37\frac{1}{2}$, (b) 187.5 or $187\frac{1}{2}$, (c) 46.875, 46.88, $46\frac{13}{15}$, or 47, (d) 225, (e) 56.25 or $56\frac{1}{4}$; (9) (a) 18.75, $18\frac{3}{4}$, or 19, (b) 93.75, $93\frac{3}{4}$, or 94, (c) 93.75 or 94; (d) 112.5 or 113, (e) 112.5 or 113; (10) (a) 43.75, $43\frac{3}{4}$, or 44, (b) 218.75 or 219, (c) 72.9, $72\frac{11}{12}$, or 73, (d) 262.5 or $262\frac{1}{2}$, (e) 87.5 or $87\frac{1}{2}$

Page 133

(1) 24 mEq, (2) 0.75 million U, (3) (a) 37.5 or 38 gtt/min, (b) 0.9 million U, (4) 16 mEq, (5) 6 mEq, (6) (a) 2.5 U, (b) 7.5 U, (7) (a) 12.5 or gtt xiii/min, (b) 4 AM, (8) (a) 6.25 g or 6250 mg, (b) 0.104 g or 104 mg, (9) 45, (10) (a) 10 ml, (b) 290 ml, (c) 116 gtt/min

Page 137

(1) 4 g, (2) 25 g, (3) 125 ml (cc), (4) 25 ml (cc), (5) 625 ml (cc), (6) 13.5 g, (7) 50 g, (8) 50 g, (9) 2.16 g, (10) 125 ml (cc), (11) 3.03 tab., (12) 20 ml (cc), (13) 15 ml (cc), (14) 40 tab., (15) 250 ml (cc), (16) 900 ml (cc) or flℨxxx, (17) 360 ml (cc) or flℨxii, (18) 10 ml, (19) 4.5 g, (20) 72 g, (21) 80 ml (cc), (22) 4.5 g, (23) 40 ml (cc), (24) 3000 ml (cc) or flℨ 100, (25) 50 ml (cc)